Alchemy for Women

Penelope Shuttle is a well-known feminist poet and novelist. She has published 5 collections of verse as well as 5 novels. Her most recent volume of poetry is **Taxing the Rain** and she is currently working on a new novel and a collection of poems.

Peter Redgrove read science at Cambridge and has worked as a research scientist and scientific journalist. He has published 23 volumes of poetry and is considered to be one of Britain's leading poets. He has also published 9 novels and 14 of his plays have been broadcast. He trained as a lay analyst with John Layard, one of Jung's pupils. Penelope and Peter live their creative life in Cornwall in accordance with the menstrual rhythms.

Together, they have collaborated on several works, including **The Wise Wound**, a groundbreaking study of the facts, fantasies and taboos surrounding the menstrual cycle. This fascinating book received wide attention when first published in 1978 and was highly praised:

'An Aladdin's cave of scientific, psychological and anthropological insights ... all quite irresistible' *The Observer*

'The first accessible book about menstruation as a human reality ... entirely praiseworthy' *Sunday Times*

'It was **The Wise Wound** that presented to a new generation of emancipated women in the 1980s what seemed at first to be a daring and paradoxical message: correctly approached and understood, menstruation need not be Woman's "curse". It can be an empowering and indeed magical experience.' Chris Knight, author of **Blood Relations: Menstruation and the Origins of Culture**

By the same authors

The Wise Wound

Alchemy for Women

Personal transformation through
dreams and the female cycle

Penelope Shuttle
& Peter Redgrove

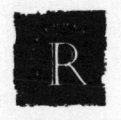

RIDER
LONDON · SYDNEY · AUCKLAND · JOHANNESBURG

This edition first published 1995

1 3 5 7 9 10 8 6 4 2

Copyright © Peter Redgrove and Penelope Shuttle 1995

The right of Peter Redgrove and Penelope Shuttle to be identified as the Authors of this work has been asserted by them in accordance with the Copyright, Designs and Patents Act, 1988.

All rights reserved. No part of this publication may be reproduced, stored in a retrieval system, or transmitted in any form or by any means, electronic, mechanical, photocopying, recording or otherwise, without the prior permission of the copyright owners.

This edition published in 1995 by Rider,
an imprint of Ebury Press, Random House,
20 Vauxhall Bridge Road, London SW1V 2SA

Random House Australia (Pty) Limited
20 Alfred Street, Milsons Point, Sydney,
New South Wales 2061, Australia

Random House New Zealand Limited
18 Poland Road, Glenfield,
Auckland 10, New Zealand

Random House South Africa (Pty) Limited
PO Box 337, Bergvlei, South Africa

Random House UK Limited Reg. No. 954009

Illustration on page 56 from **Woman's Mysteries** by M. Esther Harding © 1971 by The C. G. Jung Foundation for Analytical Psychology. Reprinted by arrangement with Shambhala Publications, Inc.

Extract on pages 103-4 from **Sex and the Brain** by Jo Durden-Smith and Diane deSimone reproduced by permission of the authors.

Papers used by Rider Books are natural, recyclable products made from wood grown in sustainable forests.

Typeset by SX Composing Ltd, Rayleigh, Essex
Printed and bound in Great Britain by Mackays of Chatham, PLC

A CIP catalogue record for this book
is available from the British Library

ISBN 0-7126-9859-0

Menstrual problems may be caused by underlying disease and if there is any suspicion of this a doctor must be consulted. The material in this book is intended for information purposes only. None of the suggestions or information is meant in any way to be prescriptive. Any attempt to treat a medical condition should always come under the direction of a competent physician – and neither the Publisher nor the Authors can accept responsibility for injuries or illness arising out of a failure by a reader to take medical advice.

*Dedicated to the women who had the courage
to tell their dreams and to live by them*

Grateful acknowledgment is due to the women and men who have given permission for their dreams to be quoted in this book.

'Out of man and woman make a round circle . . . and you will have the philosopher's stone.'

The Rosary of the Philosophers

Contents

Introduction: Scrim   1

Part I: Eve's Dream
1. The Joy of Dreaming   9
2. The Road of Trials   16
3. Dream-blood   25

Part II: Hints to Dreamers
4. The Menstrual Mandala: the Cycle at a Glance   31
5. Dream-rhythms   38
6. Some Warnings and Encouragements   46
7. Men and Menstruation   66

Part III: Further Practices
8. Moon and Weather   77
9. A Note on Rhythm   87
10. Discarding the Negative   91
11. Brain Opposites   96
12. Beyond Logic: the Right Brain   106
13. The Two Cycles   114
14. Rites of Passage   119
15. A Useful Waking-dream Technique   121
16. Yoga and its Analogues   127
17. Homeopathy, Hypnosis, Acupuncture and Massage   146
18. Relaxation Practice Outline   151

Afterword: Towards a Summary   154
Appendix: Various Dreamers', Experience of the Cycle   157
Notes   170
Bibliography of Works Cited   174

Introduction: Scrim

Scrim is the fine open-weave fabric which is used in the theatre for transformation scenes. Lighted from the front, scrim looks opaque, depressing. Light it from behind and it becomes transparent, revealing depth upon depth of magical scenery.

This is like a depression vanishing. Something almost unimaginable is going on behind the appearance of things.

You may have seen a very popular series of books called *Magic Eye*. These contain computer-generated images which look like repetitious rags and fragments if you inspect them with a hard, inquisitorial eye. Allow the gaze to soften, and the flat surface deepens miraculously, and there, so solid that you cannot believe they have not been visible all along, are radiant, almost psychedelic images. Accompanying this is a pleasant sensation, like meditation; of things coming together and making sense.

Behind the over-busy, opaque, depressing scrim of modern life there are two things which can light up the scene, depth upon depth. They have been neglected and repressed because that policy suits the controllers of power. These two things are free, profoundly liberating and deeply individual: they are *dreaming* and the rhythmic *cycle of women*.

Most people live hidden in the scrim, and the lights do not go on inside their world. Dreams, however strange and gorgeous, are disregarded. Many women who are mothers live a life of busking or quick-change artistry. A recent television commercial illustrated this tellingly. A wife and mother becomes, in response to the day's events, clown, schoolmistress, nurse, cordon bleu chef, conjurer, mime artist and, at bathtime, frogwoman. Moreover, for many women, this busking is accomplished under the shadow of menstrual distress. This further fragments their world. What 'magic eye' will change a two-dimensional world to 3-D, reconcile all these rags and fragments so that things come together and make sense?

1

This 'magic eye' exists. It is *dreaming with the cycle*. The dream cycle *is* the menstrual cycle.

The female cycle is not just a physical or physiological matter, it is also accompanied by spiritual events – that is, dreams. The dreams, if you like, are the meanings of cycle-events. It is as though these cycle-events – ovulation, pre-menstruation, menstruation, pre-ovulation – are symbolic of something that has been neglected, and the dreams as they occur are living illustrations of this further meaning. It follows that these dreams, once contacted, are the source of a feminine sense of reality which is otherwise missing from our lives. To recover full dreaming ability is like the wonderful transformation scenes revealed behind the scrim: collective images – heroines, gods, goddesses – come out and tread the boards, mingling with the people from our ordinary lives, all transformed in the rotation of the cycle. Depressions and anxieties are experienced as crossing dream thresholds as the cycle turns from menstrual to ovulatory to menstrual again. *Menstrual distress appears to be at a minimum when dreaming is at a maximum.* This community of dreams, waking life and the cycle is the foundation of a woman culture both as up-to-date and as ancient as dreaming itself.

In order to chart and understand these dreams, we can use the *Menstrual Mandala* (see Chapter 4). 'Mandala' means 'circle' or 'wheel'; it is the wheel-cross, the earliest image known to archaeologists.

Each person's cycle is as individual as DNA, but just as all DNA is built on the double-helix pattern, so each monthly cycle resembles a turning wheel. There is at one and the same time a cycle-structure of the dream, and a dream-structure of the cycle.

The mandala enables you to tune into the dreams by knowing the menstrual cycle days, and to tune into the menstrual cycle days by going deeply into the dreams. This way, the quality of both dreams and cycle days will deepen.

The menstrual cycle is perhaps the most delicate and powerful instrument of self-expression that has ever existed. At ovulation, people can be created; at menstruation, a series of processes are initiated which work towards personal evolution and creative self-development. Ovulation brings you face to face with the possibilities of your own dynasty; menstruation brings you face to face with your self at its deepest levels.

INTRODUCTION

Menstruation itself has been regarded as a sickness, a curse, ever since men took charge of women's matters. Men, it is obvious, do not menstruate. They have therefore treated the process with amazement, puzzlement and suspicion. On the one hand, it is somehow godlike and has to do with resurrection: 'They bleed, they are wounded, yet they live on!' On the other hand, it is something loathsome, unclean, excremental, vampire-like. Masculine power-politics requires that opposing forces should not become too powerful. The rhythm of the feminine cycle has remained a subversive presence.

However, very many women – perhaps as many as 75 per cent – experience the anxiety and depression, the bloating, the clumsiness and confusion of thought, the skin irritations, the explosive temper, the crying, the forgetfulness, the cravings, dizziness, fatigue, palpitations and all the other symptoms which have been incorporated into the so-called pre-menstrual syndrome (PMS), and which many medical and psychological authorities offer women as the inevitable state of their womanhood.[1] Such symptoms can take up a full fortnight of a woman's cycle – roughly half a life-time in the fertile years. A doctor's first prescription for PMS may be 'Have a child'. His second, after the children have come and gone, a hysterectomy. Yet the menstrual state can be a life-enhancing, creative experience. Women who develop in accord with it have inner resources that enable them to avoid the 'empty nest' syndrome when the children are gone. There are many indications that women who study and accept their menstrual cycle pass more easily through the menopause than those who neglect it.

So why is this advantageous menstrual state guarded by such an ordeal, as if by dragons? Even women who undergo PMS greet the menstrual experience itself, when the period begins, with a wonderful sense of relief and amazement. Finding out what exactly these dragons are is a large part of the battle, but fighting naturally creates stress. And PMS symptoms are predominantly symptoms of stress.

Most of the psychological and medical literature until recently has concentrated on the negative events in the cycle. Yet a group of women asked to concentrate on positive events reported the following as characteristic of the menstrual (and sometimes the pre-menstrual) state: (1) increased creativity (well-defined as 'a continuous process of bringing forth a changing vision of oneself, and of oneself in relation to the world'); (2) the senses intensified 'like an overwhelming rush of colours, sounds and other sensations'; (3) heightened emotions; (4) thought processes which become instinctive, seem to be experienced physically: 'the split between oneself and the physical environment disappears'; (5) increased sexual awareness; (6) visionary or ecstatic states of reverie or meditation.[2]

These are sometimes called 'right-brain' abilities (see Chapter 11). If they do not take bold possession of these positive events, it is as if women are losing not only half their menstrual cycle, but half their brain as well!

The pre-menstrual state can be a gathering-up of energy and a sweeping away of preconceptions so that the woman may enter, as it were, this other house. Many of the preconceptions which are swept away indeed have to do with the idea of women's sole role as mother, or ovulator. But there are these two balanced roles, one belonging to ovulation, and the other, less familiar (and therefore stressful in approaching) belonging to menstrual events.

It is usually argued that PMT and POS (pre-ovulation syndrome, usually less severe) are purely medical problems to be treated by the mechanical administration of drugs and hormones. Medical people who take this view will also admit that the cure is uncertain, that the symptoms often recur, and the cause is unknown. It is argued by others that PMT is purely psychological, and studies are cited that purport to show that the administration of an inactive substance (placebo) is as effective as any of the remedies.

Most authorities seem to have missed the point by plumping for *either* body *or* mind as the cause. Mind and body in our daily common-sense life are two aspects of the one thing. We move from one to the other as part of living, sometimes most aware in our bodies, sometimes in our feelings, sometimes thinking, sometimes intuiting. To treat either body or mind in isolation simply makes matters worse.

A well-known chemical remedy such as Vitamin B6 may relieve a person's monthly suffering for a while, then, without apparent cause, it may cease to do so. Have the laws of biochemistry somehow been broken? The answer is to look for the mental event complementary to the physical relief. With the administration of B6, dream-recall increases. But how many GPs recommend their PMT patients to record their dreams? Nevertheless, if you are dreaming vividly, your PMS (or POS) is likely to be at a minimum.

It is almost as though the disturbing dreams of the pre-menstrual time are a substitute for the body's disorders. Or, to put it another way, if the dreams which clear the passage from the ovulatory state to the menstrual state and back again are repressed, they will come out in symptoms of stress. If the dreams are not used, they will go away, and the symptoms return.

The placebo result too can be seen in whole-person mind–body terms. Giving a placebo is a ritual act. An accredited person in the healer's uniform of a white coat gives a person a 'magic' pill. If there is an active medicine in the pill, its effect will be enhanced by the circumstances in which it is administered. If the pill is merely sugar, these circumstances will nevertheless arouse the healing powers by psychosomatic (body–mind) means. Ritual healing by the spirit, by 'magic', by right-brain action, by the use of symbols, has immemorially been the province of women. It is therefore no surprise that the 'placebo' response is effective in menstrual distress. The shame is that this response has not been more widely recognized for what it is, and that conventional science will not accept such cures as objectively 'real'. Instead we are told, 'It's all in the mind.' Nothing human can be 'all in the mind'.

Woman-culture, we believe, is being dreamed again by contemporary women. PMS and pre-ovulatory distress seem to be at least partly due to the non-acceptance and repression of powerful female, cycle-oriented dreaming. There are two conditions in which menstrual distress tends to be at a minimum: when a person is confident in her dreams, is relating them to the cycle, and is dreaming freely; and when she has solidarity with other women with whom she can compare these feminine experiences and realities of the cycle, for it is likely that the attitudes and even the presence of men, whose hormonal constitution tends to resist the rhythms of women, are also a cause of menstrual distress.

So why 'Alchemy'? The old alchemists thought there was a philosopher's stone that would turn base metal to gold. Their fascinating texts in which blood is equated with gold, are written in a kind of dream double-speak for the transformations and distillations of the menstrual cycle. The double-speak conceals that it was an art practised by and for women, though men with careful study could partake of these transformations. Much that is needed for this study will be found in this book. We are showing here – perhaps for the first time in this age – how the cycle's apparent vagaries and inconsistencies are the product of imposed values in which the cycle has lost its balance for most people. We show how the dream-structure of the cycle is answered by the cycle-structure of the dream, and how artificial torsions result in a falsifying of the personality.

Women are by nature the strongest dreamers.

Part I

Eve's Dream

'The Dreamer is the person responsible for the continued existence of the people as a psychic (that is, tribal) entity. It is through her dreams that the people have being; it is through her dreams that they find ways to function in whatever reality they find themselves ... the Dreamer, who is the mother of the people not because she gives physical birth ... but because she gives them life through her power of dreaming.'

Paula Gunn Allen, *The Sacred Hoop* (1986)

1. The Joy of Dreaming

'Staying in a fashionable house, rather untidy, I take a wireless to be repaired. As I hand it to repair man my sanitary towel falls to the ground. I swoop down to pick it up but blood is pouring out of me. This seems suddenly very funny.' [Day 30]

'Kept laughing in this dream at funny names. I was lying on the jetty, warm boards. The name of a man, ADJUSTANCE TROUSERS, makes me laugh.' [Day 6]

'In a group of men and women, being pursued. We all hide in a room, I in a wardrobe. When it seems our pursuers have gone, we emerge, I go to the toilet, a large bathroom. Through a window I look up and see the leader of our pursuers. He sees me and again we're pursued. We all come to a shore, are rescued by men, navy? A cruiser is going to take us away. I see a smaller boat – it has "paraffin" written on it. I know it will collide with the cruiser – it does – there is an explosion – we all laugh it is so funny.' [Day 28]

Eve wakes laughing. Dreams *are* funny, more often than not. Anything as mentally agile, vivid, transformative, energetic as a good dream ought to bring laughter. Why were dreams ever thought to be obscure? They are to be enjoyed. Is a birthday present obscure? It's something you are given to wear, or play with, or exchange for something better, or to show love. Dreams are like this and, like presents, give energy, stimulate giving. Dreams most resemble the interesting and good things of life. You can wake laughing at a dream, and feel cheerful all that day. So why are they thought so obscure, wrapped about with gloomy systems of interpretation, with censors and psychiatrists? They belong to all, volatile and amusing as water, taking every shape, refreshing. No wonder every sleeping dreamer is found by research to be sexually aroused![1]

The answer is probably that the psychology of dreams is a male preserve, and men are actually not very good dreamers. This, you may say, is ludicrous: why should the power of cultural interpretation be given over to the people who, by and large, are not very expert with the basic materials? Yes, it is foolish, but the time has come when the visionaries – women – having found that men cannot make much of such gifts, must show by example what dreaming is all about. We have been taught not to believe in our dreams. The dream-environment has been polluted by misdirections. Dream is imagination, and imagination is life.

'I am riding on something which is half-bike, half-horse. Prince Charles is beside me explaining the gears. We go into a castle, up mossy stone steps, where the Queen greets us. I go through massive rooms, making for oak door marked LADIES and follow some women in. [This is a woman's dream that came with her period.] The figure of Prince Charles had a humorous and friendly feeling. He was a sort of Green Engineer, adjusting my horse for me. The dream was more enjoyable, though, when he was left behind, with his half-mechanical horse. But he was out of place and I felt safer in the castle. I was going somewhere where no man is meant to follow, both in the dream – the Ladies – and in outer reality too because I had my period. That the period was more important to me than simply a matter of slipping the gears was plain because the Queen was there. Prince Charles is an advocate of global contraception measures. I'm quite sure my horse would not like that, nor being turned into machinery. My castle at that time was my nature as a woman.

'The dream makes fun of Prince Charles, one's waking self may think unjustly, but the dream is very direct. He is a very interesting character, dream-wise. A royal male is supposed to be a kind of stallion, siring a dynasty. Charles indeed has done his part in this, but he is interested in things outside "ovulism". He is interested in the environment, the field of forces in which we live, he is interested in imaginative matters, and talks to flowers. So my dream takes him part-way along the path to the Ladies, with his interesting, fiddling little invention. That is how my dream sees it, anyway.'

It's the case that the 'play' with the dream can be interpreted along other ideological routes, but this was one which satisfied and interested the dreamer and went along with the release, by the natural bleeding, of some pre-menstrual tension. Did the dream release the tension, or the tension create the dream? Why decide that point? Does it matter? The physical release was accompanied by an amusing mental picture, and the one helped the other; perhaps the tension was caused in the delicate pre-menstrual time by some irritation with the male view of things, disguised as a logical proposition. In fact, it is a good general rule: 'When there is dreaming, menstrual tension or distress is at a minimum.'

It is remarkable that people do not consider dreams to be a playful use of energy, will not play with them, question and answer. If you do, their humour and vividness will escalate, and you will notice fresh images and fresh standpoints. (But perhaps that is how *women* approach dreams anyway, if they are not told otherwise.)

Another remarkable thing about dreams is that the so-called experts have not seen fit to comment that much of the imagery of dreams demonstrates the menstrual cycle. That is to say, the series of events which constitute the cycle are supported by vivid dreaming germane to those bodily events. In men this is also the case, as they respond to the menstrual cycle of the women they live with, or have lived with (the mother, for instance). No wonder men have been puzzled by dreams, since they have no cycle of their own.

This fact, already known to many women, was first established many years ago by the researches of Therese Benedek and Boris Rubenstein.[2] Since then the matter has occasionally been revisited by other workers, and each time the study has been made this same fact has emerged. Yet the significance to women of this discovery has been repeatedly allowed to drop out of sight.

There is generation, and there is regeneration. Or call them ovulation, and menstruation. There is the ovulation domain in our lives, and the menstruation domain. These are the sources of the deepest conflict in lives and societies. Ovulation is the generation of loved children. Menstruation is a flood of personal creativity.

You can see this in the dreams. Dreams in the menstrual domain are characteristically about primitive and powerful unexpected experiences.

'*I go to the bathroom and find that my period has started*

unexpectedly early. I see that sperms are among the blood. Later I check again and see that the sperms have developed and grown, which must mean that I am pregnant. The next time I check I find, instead of blood, drawings on the toilet tissue. They are drawings I had done years ago and had completely forgotten. They depict either an evolutionary process or the growth of a child to adulthood. It is the development of small, stooped mankind to man in an upright posture. The last picture is that of prehistoric woman holding the hand of a child. She is a lovely woman and wears just a loincloth. It reminds me of prehistoric man first discovering fire.'

Max Zeller comments:

> Out of her menstrual blood arises images, and images are the language of the soul, giving psychic meaning to the menses... It is as if the dream is in open opposition to the modern outlook that denies any special attention to the menses beyond the physiological fact ... she receives and conceives images from the dark transpersonal realm and gives them back by reflecting and writing and painting. The child that will be born from this union is not a physical child; it is non-corporeal; its nature will be spiritual.[3]

On the other hand the emblems in dreams at ovulation tend to be intimate and close to more tender feelings: 'Somebody bought me a beautiful pearl earring, just one.' This ovulation dream of a precious object held in the ear, analogue of the Fallopian tube, occurred on Day 14, a usual day for ovulation. Brenda Mallon in her *Women Dreaming*[4] quotes some beautiful ovulation dreams.

One of her subjects, in a dream, was holding and looking at small, delicate and beautifully-wrought objects, jewellery especially. She dreamed of cut-glass jewels which were tiny multicoloured cubes in her hand. She took off some green alabaster scarab earrings to find that one of them had cracked into four pieces though it remained in the setting. Brenda Mallon points out that fertilized eggs divide first into two, then into four, and so on. She says: 'It is as if Kate's dream continues that natural development in symbolic form.'

Green is also a colour associated with ovulation. The scarab

THE JOY OF DREAMING

beetle, rolling its spheres of food for its larvae, was to the ancient Egyptians an image of the powers behind the cycle. The scarab is also said to have twenty-eight joints to its body. According to the Jungian writer Marie Louise Von Franz, green things are of Osiris, red things of Seth, the 'antagonist'. This ancient Egyptian tradition reflects today, as it did in the long past, a self-division forced on women.

Therese Benedek[5], one of the few psychologists to relate dreams to the cycle systematically (Havelock Ellis was another), also found in the 1930s that dreams of precious gems, and round, fragile objects were common during ovulation. She also records green dreams, including one of a dinosaur: 'very slimy and shining and ugly green.' This can be read as the awakening of ovulatory energy in a patient who feared ovulation as a monstrous interference with her personal life.

One very beautiful ovulation dream reported to ourselves concerned a single round and flashing diamond earring, as it might be the egg entering the Fallopian tube. Dreams of birds' eggs are also frequent, as are round forms like tables, even the Round Table of King Arthur as the whole cycle seen at ovulation (Barbara Walker says the original setting had twenty-eight seats).[6] One woman who turned into a powerful and glittering 'Mrs Wonderful' at ovulation dreamed of a great flashing, dazzling shield inset with mirrors, like some glittering device to fascinate the little sperm-birds.

Another woman's dream seemed to reflect the egg's implantation: a shuttle-craft was docking on to a much larger mother-ship, astronauts were steering it in with careful gestures and radioed instructions: 'Up a bit. Just a little to your left.' That shuttle-craft is now our daughter, aged seventeen, and experiencing her cycle with remarkable dreams.

The pattern of withdrawal and return (with the treasure hard to find), made famous by Joseph Campbell in his book *The Hero with a Thousand Faces*, very likely originated in the female monthly cycle, and was then taken over by the male. *The Hero with a Thousand Faces* must one day be rewritten by one of these female heroes, or heras. The 'treasure hard to find' is either a physical child or a spiritual–magical one.

The journey is less perilous for one who knows her own rhythms, who is in tune with them, and does not want a child, not this cycle, anyway. Brenda Mallon quotes another beautiful dream about journeys. There were trains and tunnels and walking across rough land. There was a rough track and a farmworker's cottage at the end of it. A man and a woman were standing in the doorway, and the woman was pregnant again, but she knew she was going to give birth to a fish this time. The dreamer watched her give birth to a long, smooth, greeny-coloured fish. It changed to a sea-green ornamental dolphin, which was beautiful, translucent and glasslike. Later the dreamer noticed that it had fallen to the floor and smashed in fragments, but this did not worry her as it was 'part of the natural order'.

This fortunate dreamer was sufficiently in touch with the natural processes not to regret the death of the ovum, and would probably not therefore suffer from PMS to any great extent, especially as she was also accustomed to dreaming. A regular dream in the post-ovulation quadrant is that one has lost one of one's existing children, sometimes violently, as from a boat or plane, sometimes by leaving them in the playground or equivalent situation. This is a difficult dream to have, but it means not hanging on to ovulatory values, as in the cycle's turning other values are revealed.

The fish is a frequent symbol of conception: either physical conception of a child at ovulation, or of a mental or spiritual conception during the period. The latter is likely to be a magical fish that talks and gives advice, like *The Magic Flounder* in the Grimm tale. In that case it will signify awareness in the womb-waters, or in the unconscious; the fish is a survivor of the mythical flood, and its eye never closes, like God's. This does not preclude a phallic connotation.

An ovulation dream of a different dreamer is recorded by Brenda Mallon. Here there is a twelve-year-old boy who has been abandoned, and a purse found in which are some semi-precious stones and a goldfish swimming around in too-little water. The dreamer wants more water for the fish. This dreamer may very well be about to enter her post-luteal or pre-menstrual phase with no conception, and one may read the mention of water as too little birth-water as she is not pregnant. She may have hydration symptoms – a symbolic attempt to save up birth-water – but probably without distress as she is a dreamer.

Dreams of water are very frequent during post-ovulation. One woman regularly dreamed that she was sloshing about in wellington boots full of water at the time when her body retained water to the extent that her rings felt tight. Another woman would always dream, post-ovulation, of a sea voyage. This same dreamer would also, month after month, dream of a rugby-game at ovulation, with two teams competing for the egg-shaped ball.

The archetypes, the great collective symbols, tend to appear in dreams if the dreamer is stressed, instead of symptoms of physical stress (PMS or POS). They reappear every month with changes of the menstrual cycle in so far as these are stressful. Such images are concerned with adult growth and psychological maturity. According to Ann Belford Ulanov:

> [The archetypes] act like magnetic fields which, though unseen, arrange responses, emotions and actions into specific patterns expressed in the form of symbolic images. If the ego can relate to these archetypal centres of energy through their symbolic expressions, the use of instinctive energy can be consciously guided for the ego's purposes.[7]

If your body generates these images in sleep, in dreams or daydreams, in approaching sleep, or coming out of it, then the channels are open. Like Alice floating down her rabbit-hole, one can descend towards the dream in ordinary nightly sleep. Alice was a man's image of how one might confront the figures of a dream – with polite affection or scornful fearlessness, like a St Joan of the Vision of the Night. It is a good attitude, but it is best to remember that one is there primarily to learn, and also that the dream-figures have feelings and thoughts, as you do, and they are part of your seeking knowledge, as is your consciousness.

The great knowledge in this context is how different ovulation and menstruation seem to each other: they are like antagonists. One must consider menstruation's view of ovulation (loss of soul in domestic bliss) and how it conflicts with ovulation's view of menstruation (child-stealer; cannibal-witch). It is the conflict between the two, paradoxical to each other, which, when healed, heals all.

2. The Road of Trials

A member of a women's group gave this account of a waking dream that opened up her whole menstrual cycle to her.

'We had been given relaxation practice, and my body inside my skin felt calm and deep. The leader now gave a suggestion: "Find yourself in a place which is the exact image of your menstrual cycle." Immediately I was in a green field which I saw was marked out in a great magic circle made of four quadrants. One quadrant was water, another was green grass, the third was a tunnel that wound in within the earth, the fourth was a series of mountain-peaks. I entered the fourth, and ascended into the mountain passes, where I met an old-young man who became my dream-counsellor for a time.'

That was a waking dream brought about by suggestion in a state of profound relaxation. It did in fact give to the waking dreamer a deep feeling for the shape of her cycle: the menstrual mandala. It is likely that she was in a late ovulation, early pre-menstrual phase. Mountain peaks can signify dangerous highs and lows in the changeover from the flooding with the pregnancy hormone progesterone at luteal phase to the later drop in its levels, before its replacement by womb neuro-transmitters and prostaglandins at menstruation. But this is medical jargon (see Chapter 13). In dream-reality, the mountains were inhabited. The old-young man, the Old Boy (title of Confucius) is a figure both of ovulation (young) and menstruation (spiritually mature) in whom opposites unite.

The ordeals are severe. Most women experience them physically, rather than making the discoveries the dream-images imply. Who can blame this majority, deprived of sister-solidarity? But as we have observed, women are by nature better dreamers than men, at least initially: women are *natural* dreamers. It is astonishing how quickly PMS can pass by encouraging and understanding the dreams.

See it as a quest. The treasure? Understanding the whole rhythm: menstruation – ovulation – menstruation – wholeness. The 'ordeals' occur at the changes of the cycle, the transitions and separations. These changes are initially unconscious because women's mysteries have been deprived of their revelance. You can see one way in which this has been done by reading the biblical prohibitions against menstruation in Leviticus.[1]

As the two great culminations – ovulation and menstruation – are so different, to change from the one to the other is a feat of transformation, a shape-shifting. So it is at these change-overs that trouble occurs. We began with ovulation, which gives rise to wonderful dreams, if, that is, ovulation is part of your temperament as it is part of our culture. This predominance of the egg will last about three days (say Days 14 to 17 in a twenty-eight day cycle) when fertilization and implantation are possible. Sexually and emotionally this can be a wonderful time. But what happens as the egg dies? Inwardly, this is like the end of the world. It is actually the beginning of another world. Reaching that other world is the way of ordeals, *separation* from ovulation and *transition* to menstruation.

Dreams that are immediately post-ovulation (separation) often, as we saw, involve ordeal by water. They are associated with the peak of the pregnancy hormone, progesterone, and may go with an actual hydration, an accumulation of water, as if to stand for birth-water. Later on, dreams nearer the period (transition) may be of ordeals of blood and fire, for example being burned as a witch. In fact they are approaching the magic fire of menstruation.

Here are some frequent images met in ovulation, early pre-menstrual and late pre-menstrual domain dreams. There is some overlapping between thresholds and domains, and, of course, a cycle does not have to be twenty-eight days long. We will return to this.

FREQUENT DREAM IMAGES IN THE OVULATION DOMAIN – DAYS 14 TO 21
Fragile precious things: jewels, eggs, fish, earrings. Round things generally: tables, footballs and football games.

Colour green. White-and-gold colours. Superwoman. Green tree. Xmas Tree. Baby. Bird.

Young children. Benevolent Jekyll. Personal Mother. Domestic animals. White wine. Double house. White chair. Feast. Butterflies.

POST-OVULATION TO EARLY PRE-MENSTRUAL – DAYS 17 TO 25. SEPARATION FROM OVULATION
Female comedians. Animals fighting. 'Jaws.' White flowers dying, red flowers blooming. Lesbian images. Yellow colours. Nasty shit. Terrible father/mother.

Malevolent Jekyll. Damaged vessels. Scarabs, beetles. Losing child. Pitcher broken. Crucifix.

Wicked ladies. Birth of feral child. Sinister church. Police. Fencing. Fight with eggs. Baby born with teeth. Green apple eaten. Golden child and or mother.

Ordeals by water: swimming pool with shark in it.

LATE PRE-MENSTRUAL – DAYS 25 TO 28.
TRANSITION TO MENSTRUATION DOMAIN
Male comedians. Red ants. Rape. Bestiality. Witch-burning. Vampires. Axe-murderer. 'Freddie' (*Nightmare on Elm Street*). Sphinx. Shit-fertile. Homosexuality. Poppies. Going into gents. Abominable meal. Brothels. Whores. Fridges. Book of magic. Passing through a small room. Initiation chamber.

Untamed feline animals. Dreamer metamorphoses into animal. Exploding animal. Red wine. Moths. Double house. Hooded dwarves. Man in black. White clothes stained or spattered red or black. Red sofa. Red coals. Petrol bursting into flames.

Man unharmed in flames, furnace. Black man. Tiles falling. Dental operations. Falling off roof. Military manoeuvres and engagements. Red wine.

Being a spy. Cleaning hearth, chimney. Benevolent Hyde. Bat. Red cakes eaten. Hospital operations. Moonlit scenes.

Bathroom between two rooms. Dirty toilets. Willing death. Ordeals by fire: burnt as a witch.

These separation and transition dreams are full of struggle and ordeal. The agonizing process reverses all the ovulation values, which are transformed to menstrual ones. The dreams are a crucible. But if the images are dreamed, the physical distress is at a minimum. It is possible to have a big separation-from-ovulation dream at around Day 21 that clears the road, does the whole job in one dream, and leaves you with a clear and energetic pre-menstrual week, with little trouble about the transition to the menstrual domain. Separation times are often associated with anxiety, and transition times sometimes carry depression with them as well. Both anxiety and depression can be dispelled by a dream which speaks out.

The Two Houses

A very frequent transition image of passing the post-ovulation threshold consciously, and therefore with more interest than distress, is that of the two houses. One is familiar, and that is the ovulation house, full of family; the other is much more dark and mysterious and contains difficult treasures, and lovers or magicians rather than husbands.

The transition between these two houses is also by an ordeal: one may have to swing out of one window and into another to get access, and one may be helped by a female friend who knows the way. Women's dreams differ quite markedly from men's in that the women have same-sex helpers, while the men tend to have a hostile relation to same-sex figures and may spend a lot of time fighting these shadows off before accepting what they offer. High places tend to signify a hormone high, and the danger here is falling off the high place and into a depression, that is (in chemical terms) falling off the oestrogen or progesterone highs before the menstrual phase has had a chance to give energy. Another frequent pre-menstrual dream is of falling off a high roof with red tiles.

Between the two houses of ovulation and menstruation, then, is a small room. One has to crawl through. Or there may be a crawlspace between floors, or a bathroom in which one is washed. Or a bedroom with two doors in which a dangerous male person sleeps, signifying the strong animus energies of the menstruation. It may be a toilet, which is likely not to be clean, and the dreamer may find herself dirtied with excrement, but may also find precious things in the bowl among the excrement.

Excremental images point to a very common childhood trauma,

which is thankfully less frequent than it used to be, at the menarche or first period. The girl has not been told what to expect when her period comes, and it arrives unawares at a most embarrassing moment, staining her clothes, as if she were incontinent. This arouses all the shames and terrors of toilet-training, which then alas become associated with menstruation. 'Official' accounts of menstruation in encyclopaedias and medical books promote the idea of menstrual blood as a kind of excrement which has no other function than to be got rid of. In fact the blood is a love-juice, equal but opposite to the white love-juice of ovulation. Prevailing social attitudes acting within the family still associate menstrual blood with shit. This gives ovulation an opportunity to despise her opposite, leading to pre-menstrual depression with a negative view as to what the menstrual time may hold in store. Hence the terrifying and terrific dream-images.

The bloody and rending images, which are so distressing, we believe relate to the giving up of the ovum to ruin and collapse, against the ovulation instinct. Sometimes this perplex has been reinforced by the fact that the clitoris becomes exceptionally sensitive pre-menstrually, and a girl may think, in bringing her first period on by masturbating, that she has injured herself. That is, if she is not prepared for the blood-flow, she believes that she has injured herself radically for pleasure, and the shame this brings becomes associated with the period. People who don't mind feeling naughty pass these thresholds with more ease: creative divergers as opposed to conservative convergers. Sexuality and climax – with its devotion, its concentration, its hurling the personality into the unknown, its re-forming after the 'little death' – is a wonderful technique for crossing dangerous thresholds. Images in reverie or dream which accompany or follow the climax come from deep down, and should be valued accordingly.

The Abominable Meal

Another terrifying frequent post-ovulatory pre-menstrual image is 'the abominable meal'. Shit is eaten, or the flesh of some repulsive animal, or a tabooed animal, or spoiled meat is eaten, or human meat, 'long pig', or the corpse of a relative. Again, ovulation is so different from menstruation that, when the egg recedes and breaks up, these persecutory fragments have to be reassembled and transformed with the release of energy. This means that a horror has to be dream-accepted, so radical is the change of attitude. It is equivalent to 'putting oneself outside the pale', that is, crossing the threshold by breaking an important taboo. Call it a transition from left-brain to whole-brain matters. The abominable meal is, if you like, the egg itself, whose energies are absorbed to give new power to the menstrual state. In ovulation's view this is cannibalism. Witches were supposed to eat children. In fact, the Wise Woman would know all about these dreams, and value them as initiatory stories. We have suggested elsewhere that such dreams were one of the foundations of witchcraft, and a source of the witch persecutions.[2] The persecutors would be dreaming too. Knowledge of the cycle values not only ovulation, but its opposite. The witches knew more of women's matters than their persecutors, who then interpreted witch practices as cannibalism and took the biblical view that ovulism was the only good. The witch-finders would be persecuted by their own fearful dreams, and react violently to them.

So dreams of being a witch – that is, knowledgeable about women's 'magic' – often arrive late in the pre-menstrual quadrant. As mentioned above, one may, especially in the fourth week, dream of the ordeal of fire, or being burned as a witch. The fire is menstrual energy, consuming the old ovulator, who emerges from the flames a new person.

Transformations

With knowledge of the dreams, the passage from ovulation to menstruation grows smoother, and the terrors ease. But until conflicts are resolved, remarkable changes are experienced: images of metamorphosis, of premature burial, of transformation in the grave to a vampire, of zombies rising from the dead.

In one woman's dream she became a dog by growing a muzzle on the top of her head and two extra eyes at the back. Her limbs rotated so that she walked on all fours, her belly where her back was.

Transformation into an animal, intercourse with an animal, or close companionship with one, means re-establishing a connection with suppressed instinctive energies in this energetic pre-menstrual quadrant. This is like a 'rite of passage' not only to the right brain, but deeper to the primitive animal brain too. It is a quest to integrate all potentialities. A dog would also symbolize acute animal non-visual senses, which increase as menstruation comes.

The Terrible Mother, the Dark Man and the Shark

Figures of the mother tend to appear late in the third week (separation from ovulation) and she comes in her terrible form, as this is the time when the womb can begin to howl its sorrow that there is no occupant. The Terrible Mother as Old Witch chases the dreamer to put her into her empty oven, since she has no baby. A mother may dream of her daughter as a young witch stealing her fertility and beauty. Daughters tend to come into their fertility when the mother is approaching menopause and is beginning to question her own fertility and ability to interest a partner. This competitive aspect of family dynamics has hardly been explored because of the taboo against all things menstrual.

Very important in the dreams moving towards menstruation are the images of black people, or marriage to a black or dark man. There are no racial connotations here; the image declares an opposite and therefore a complement. There is marriage to one's own dark side, certainly, and sacred or transpersonal incest, as it signifies the incorporation of sensuous experiences first encountered in early childhood, unseen, invisible, dark, active at night. More directly than that, 'blackness' in this context among white people signifies the non-visual senses. We would hope that data will be gathered of the corresponding dream opposites in black people. Traditional African spirit- and dream-folk are often visualized as being white.

Peter Redgrove argued in *The Black Goddess* that the visual senses are the 'high' or 'theoretical' senses, associated with intellect, detachment and 'scientific' manipulation of the outer world. We have seen how our own society is concerned with display and outer meaning as opposed to subjectivity and inner meaning. The whole data of science are read off visually on instruments which indicate by pointers, numbers and VDUs. Visualization is the chief tool of abstract intellect. The 'dark' or 'animal' senses, by contrast, involve one's own self and known and trusted people within an intimate space. A small, dark or cramped room is a frequent dream image for entering the menstrual state; but it is ovulation's cramping view of the menstrual experience, which later opens out.

Just as the emphasis tends to shift from left brain to right brain during the passage from ovulation to menstruation, so the sensory modalities tend to shift towards the non-visual state. A Black Goddess then becomes the symbol of this transformation, with black men as her messengers.

Marilyn Nagy-Bond has shown that, in her group of women, images of the Strange Man and of the Mother dominated dreaming at the menses or thereabouts.[3] We have noticed that the Terrible Mother attends the immediately post-ovulatory ordeal by water much more often than she did before the film *Jaws*. This image has gained focus as a shark, haunting swimming-pools or other bodies of water through which the dreamer has to pass. The clear water may be stained with human blood, the dreamer becomes a spectator of her ovulation world where even her children are slaughtered. Later the dreamer may find herself passing through the water quite safely, able to breathe it, like a fish. If this happens it shows a great familiarity with the passage through this threshold, amounting to a rebirth, for the shark symbolizes among other things the perils of rebirth, the destroying womb of the mother, echoed in the dreamer's own womb-blood.

Since the menstrual blood and its smell are associated with the first occasion on which we smelled blood, that is, our births, then it is a doorway to the recovery of energies caught up in the birth-trauma. If the dreamer reports being conscious of the dark senses, being able to *touch* and *taste* in these dreams and, most particularly, *smell*, then one may expect profound transformations. These are the senses involved in the multimedia show of birth. Visual images are less immediate here; the child does not form them until later. As the senses are not so separated out at birth, the experience would incorporate enormous flashes of light and dark, and deafening noises, in which the safe and knowledgeable events would be the smell, taste and touch of the mother. This is the rebirthing power of the non-visual.

The hormones of the mother are increased greatly at birth, and the foetus is affected by them into a kind of tumescence of the whole body. Passage down the birth-canal with all its squeezing and massage is like an orgasm of the whole body. The ability to sense in this way is the 'orgasmic capacity' in the adult, and the menstrual state is one of its doorways. Hence the importance of such dreams, and also their traumatic power.

Everybody has these dreams of the menstrual cycle, men included, once they begin to look. Most will admit to the familiar ovulation dreams. The unpleasant dreams of the pre-menstrual time will be noted with interest by women tired of recurring PMS. These dreams are as accessible as the ovulation ones to all who wish to taste transformation, though transitions are tougher due to menstrual neglect.

3. Dream-blood

Just as well-established, once people start comparing notes, are the dreams heralding menstruation itself. Blood or red flowers are explicit and usual. The whole transition may be shown in images, as in the dream of one woman who reported on Day 16:

'Then I'm by the winter flowerbed full of dead flowers, and I see that the deep red geranium is beginning to flower and I am very pleased. I pick off the dead flowerheads and dead twigs, to give the red plant a good chance to flower more.'

This is a woman who has been sterilized, and in whom ovulation is no longer as significant as it once was. Women who are fertile, who have determined to have no more children but who have to struggle with their emotions and instincts regarding them at ovulation, sometimes have dreams that remind them of compensating menstrual interests at the time of ovulation. Thus one woman dreams at ovulation of an 'interesting' pregnant woman and of herself as being pregnant in the latter half of a dream, the earlier part of which showed her in a small room writing the name of a church on a mirror, to the dictation of children. Seeing the mirror-church as the 'other house', and the reversal through the mirror that would come in the change from one brain-side to another, pleased the woman and assisted the post-ovulation separation. The previous month at ovulation she had in a dream worn a black dress that glistened as with magical skin-awareness and had been shown witches as women of power.

Frequent images heralding the flow are: the wearing of red clothes, a roof of straw or rushes through which rain comes, red flowers plucked and smelled (the smelling signifies a particularly happy arrival of the period), Dracula as a lover, red mice or ants, aboriginal lovers. One woman reported: 'I don't have "nightmares" at the onset of menstruation, but tend to dream of warm red rooms richly hung with red silks.'

With the beginning of the period the non-visual senses become more wakeful, and while one woman said her body could feel for the moon more than before, another had a waking dream of a red colour and a white mist linked with her breathing.

On the night before her period, this dreamer also dreamed:

I was sitting at my desk, a small nuclear bomb in my hands. I split it in two and take out the centre, the timing mechanism. I bite this and crunch it, eat it like a nut. Then I throw the now harmless halves away into my neighbour's garden.

She effectively defused a potentially explosive conflict between the two halves of her cycle by finding the centre and treating it as sensual sustenance.

Another woman dreamed of the new crescent of the moon the night it came into the sky, and her period came too. She dreamed:

Seeing the new moon. I tell someone to take off his glasses to see it. I say, look how close Venus is to it. We look into the dark blue sky to see the moon and the star and then suddenly there are about half a dozen very bright stars that shoot into view and stay very bright for a while. We are amazed.

Day 3 is a royal occasion for this woman:

Outside in a lovely big garden park with husband, wandering and enjoying the vivid green grass, leaves, bright flowers and flowery garden smells, bright but not garish colour. We are summoned into a house. Many people. To our surprise, awe, we are in the Queen's house. Many royals are there, and we are invited to a party. Diana comes in and asks us, me, to help her with a poem she is trying to write, love poem to her husband Charles. It is a bad poem, has gaps in it. She is older, not very pretty, with a blackish stubble on her chin, powdered over. I say, you must write many descriptions of your husband, describe all you like best about him. She seems satisfied. Conversation all around, vivacious. Then I have a quite big red car that the Queen has instructed I be given.

A woman who was a practical user of the menstrual mandala – she used it to index her dreams and as a way of seeing the whole cycle at once – recorded the following images dreamed in the menstrual domain (Days 1 to 7) over several cycles:

Gift of a purple suit, purple velvet, costing £300.
Tomatoes in the outhouse, with red flowers on.
Picking a rose, carrying it into the kitchen.
Riding on a half-bike, half-horse, with Prince Charles beside me explaining the gears. We go in castle, up mossy stone steps, where the Queen greets us. I go through massive rooms, making for oak door marked LADIES *and follow some women in.*
Looking at early maps of the world.
Green roof of straw or rushes through which rain comes.
One of us has to die, it is the policy, he is a youngish blackbearded man, like a combination of D. H. Lawrence and Lenin; he is in a pinewood coffin on a trestle and is just peeping out of the lid which he lifts, saying goodbye to his wife, both weeping. But it is in a good cause. The lid is put down on him.
In a shop, mostly handbags on sale. There is a flood of water and vomit everywhere. I feel I have done it. There is an oldish woman with red hair who asks me to go with her.
Dad gives me a bottle of red wine. A good year, my mother says.
Festival. Cakes. We throw cakes at an altar.
Our kitten was run over, blood on fur.

Interpreting dreams associated with the cycle becomes natural once the connections are seen. There is a vocabulary of dreaming that develops with the person, a vocabulary which incorporates feed-back, in that the waking use of it and interest in it focuses and redefines the dreaming. The inborn collective vocabulary shows the way to redefine one's self-images. It has been said that: 'The point is that the dream should not be interpreted in terms of ordinary reality, but rather, this reality in terms of the dream.'[1] This should go both ways. Actuality and dream interact. No reality can remain 'ordinary' if it is illuminated by its dream. No dream can remain fantasy while grounded in actuality. Actuality is the spirit of the dream; dream is actuality's soul. Both dream and actuality are real.

FREQUENT DREAM IMAGES DURING MENSTRUATION

Red tree. Red clothes: scarlet to purple. Blood-red snake. Red roses plucked and smelled. Tomatoes sliced. Pomegranate. Women engaged in common purpose. Early maps. Magic tools. Black and gold. Giving birth to oneself. Horned God. Serpent. Breathing underwater. Solidarity with women. Lesbian imagery. Kind fox helping dog. Transformatory potion.

Part II

Hints to Dreamers

'Mandala: A pattern which is effective in connecting one part of experience with another, and the contemplation of which leads to insight. A mandala has a centre, a boundary or circumference, and cardinal points. It often depicts a rhythm, which one can see at a glance in a single image. The simplest form is that of the wheeled cross, and this is the most ancient symbol known. The moon cycle, with cardinal points at full and new, first and last quarter, forms just such a mandala. The menstrual cycle can take a similar shape, with menstruation and ovulation, and the start of pre-ovulation and premenstruation, as its cardinal points.'

Penelope Shuttle and Peter Redgrove, *The Wise Wound* (1994)

4. The Menstrual Mandala: The Cycle at a Glance

The menstrual mandala is the menstrual cycle's 'organizer'. It is a map for discovering and representing the shape of the period. It can be one's compass, astrolabe, talisman and moon-sextant. It takes the measure of the ups and down of the period. It is a reliable weather-forecast.

Most menstrual charts are linear. But why straighten out what is a *cycle* and therefore round, or spiral? Why not express the female rhythm in a way closer to the manner in which it arrives, a circling rhythm?

Undoubtedly this is a political matter. Linear time is a mark of masculine time – call it *Chronos*. *Kairos* is the feminine time, eternally recurring and visiting its origins. In linear time you have one chance at everything, in circular time you revisit what is important. In linear time in Christianity there is one Creation, one Fall, one Incarnation, one Day of Judgment, and this scheme of every moment representing a last chance produces anxiety, no doubt contributing among women to menstrual distress.

The unchanging sun, moving to its height in summer and its low in winter, is an image for the masculine world of unchanging ego-life. The sun's disc is never diminished, except rarely by eclipses. This is like the unvarying glare of too-masculine or left-brain consciousness. The moon winds on its labyrinthine course, waxing and waning, seemingly lost to be found again, always changing position. That is lunar time. Lunar and solar calendars don't fit together, as you will find when you embark on the year's menstrual calendar.

Professor W. M. O'Neill says of our calendar: 'What a strange hodge-podge in which nothing quite fits anything else! The weeks don't quite fit the months of the year; to make the months fit the year real Moon periods are abandoned; the years are never exact

ALCHEMY FOR WOMEN

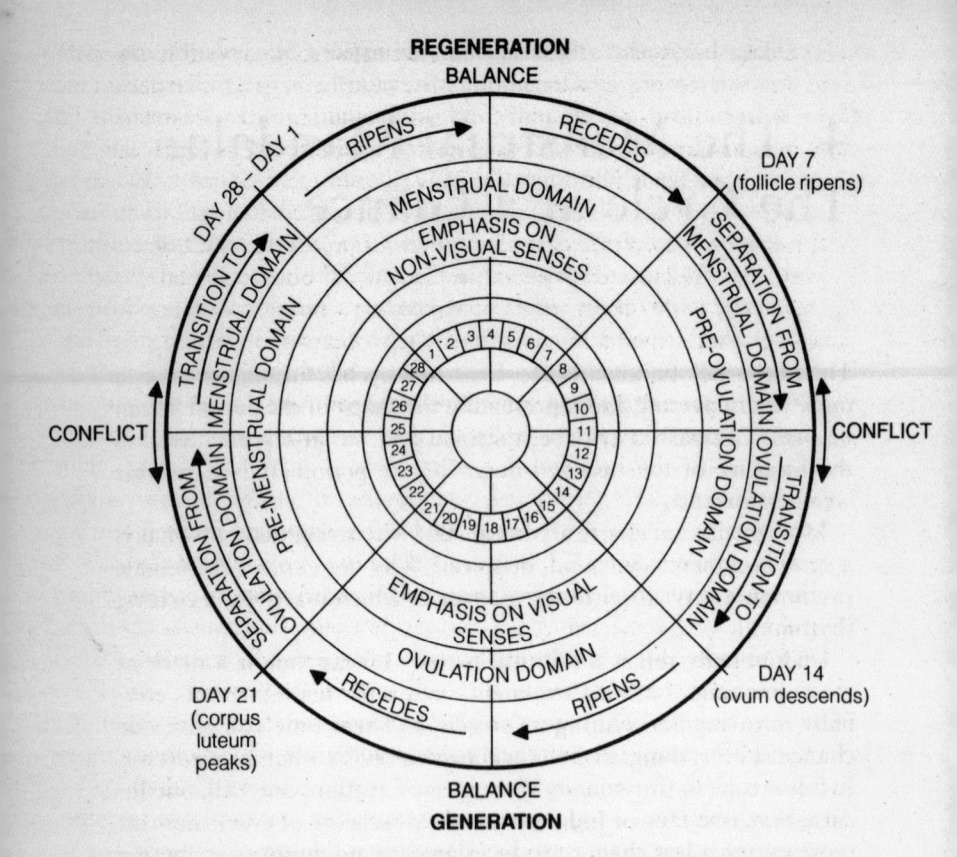

Figure 1. *The Mandala of the Menstrual Cycle*

Supposing we start at the top of the picture, menstruating at a *balance*-point. The period has ripened, it will shortly recede. If you like the period, as it recedes, conflict may begin. On Day 7, as the follicle starts its action, there may be a distinct sensation of *separation* from the period, and approaching an entirely different mode, ovulation. This conflict and *transition* to the ovulation may bring a distinct feeling of illness (mittelschmerz) which passes as you go into the ovulation and find the *balance* of pure ovulation. This recedes, and feelings of conflict arise again, particularly as the egg breaks up, releasing its energies, while the corpus luteum with its pregnancy hormone is still at its peak. This *separation* from the ovulation domain is one variety of PMS (late luteal dysphoria); the other is the *transition* to the menstrual domain again. If you can pass these separation and transition thresholds consciously and with knowledge, PMS and mittelschmerz will be at a minimum. Feed-back with the cycle events and the dreams will deepen. Twenty-eight days is an average monthly cycle, which of course varies with the individual.

solar tropical periods.'[1] There is a conflict between solar and lunar time, social time and menstrual time: it would be better for society if the women in it had a monthly five-day weekend for menstruation. Menstruation rhythm is real time felt by the body, as much as summer or winter is felt. Barbara G. Walker says:

> It has been shown that calendar consciousness developed first in women, because of their natural menstrual body calendar, correlated with observations of the moon's phases. Chinese women established a lunar calendar 3000 years ago, dividing the celestial sphere into 28 stellar 'mansions' through which the moon passed. Among the Maya of central America, every woman knew 'the great Maya calendar had first been based on her menstrual cycles'.[2]

So for real womanly time, one should make a menstrual clock – as we say, a menstrual mandala.

The basic menstrual clock-dial we recommend is very simple. With a pair of compasses, draw two small circles, one inside the other. The outer circle will be used to number the days in the calendar month, and the inner one your own personal days of the cycle. Then, according to your choice you have as many circles as you like in which you can compare the events of the month in which you are interested. Draw in the twenty-eight radii of the stack of circles – these are the cycle days.

You start filling in the mandala on the first day of your period, which is Day 1. If you have a rough idea of your cycle length, it is easy to space the days. We suggest marking crosswise the four main thresholds: that is, menstruation to pre-ovulation; pre-ovulation to ovulation; ovulation to pre-menstrual; pre-menstrual to menstrual. Or, to put it another way, mark the first day of each of the four weeks, assuming it is going to be a twenty-eight-day cycle. If it is not 'regular' then make an approximation. You can be confident that body and chart will interact and make a four-fold pattern, naturally quartering the circle.

It can be described more technically: that is, from menstrual and post-menstrual to proliferative and follicular (when the womb-wall regenerates and the ovum begins to grow fully in the ovary), then to ovulation itself, and the luteal phase and secretory stage of the womb-wall; from ovulation to recession of the corpus luteum and the pre-menstrual time. In practice most people can feel all these changes, once they are aware of what is going on. In this the menstrual mandala is a tuning device focused on natural happenings.

If you don't already know your cycle well, then it is worth learning by experience how the days arrange themselves. We have in fact drawn the cervix at the centre of our diagram; it is, you might say, the hub of the wheel.

It is a good thing to be aware of one's ovulation. Some people recognize it by ovulatory distress (of course this should be marked on the mandala); others by a few pains in the lower back or groin and a clear or even glittering, stretchy, vaginal secretion (Spinnbarkheit). Some may choose to watch the position and appearance of the cervix, using a speculum, to get an accurate view of what is going on. People using natural family planning methods will note the rise in temperature just after ovulation.

Others may want to guess that ovulation occurs just about midcycle, and they may have this confirmed by quite definite dreams. It is usually said that the post-ovulatory time is an invariable fifteen days, which is the cycle time of the ovary's corpus luteum, but this is by no means always so. Anything and everything about the cycle may vary according to who you are and what happens to you, and it may be that you linger for longer in the post-ovulatory phase than you do in the pre-ovulatory. Thresholds expand and contract according to life-events. It will be easy to see this on the mandala as days crowd into the space before either of the two culminations. Many find that a mandala not only expresses order, it creates it. Making such a pattern can indeed regularize the cycle.

You can mark cycle-days, then, in the first concentric circle moving outward. In the next circle after that, the calendar day seems the most appropriate. In the next circle you could mark negative or unpleasant symptoms (your doctor would look for the recurrence of these when diagnosing PMS). In the next largest circle after this, why not record positive symptoms and good times? If there is not enough space, use a method of coding it to the journal in which you keep your dream-record (see below). As an example, you could put the moon and weather in another circle, but there is no limit to the circles you can chart if you want to.

One of the circles could be used for marking temperature, if you are trying for a natural fertility chart. You may be using a computerized thermometer for this. The cycle responds well at first to this machine, for charting temperature with it can regularize the cycle for a brief time. Eventually, however, the cycle may grow to dislike the thermometer, and show apparently arbitrary rises. Again, these may make sense when related to other events on the menstrual mandala.

Another circle could be used for notes about dream-images. The actual dream would be written out in a dream-journal, indexed to the mandala by cycle-days. One is likely to find that negative symptoms rise when dreams disappear, but dreams often tend to disappear when waking days have been more than usually good and creative.

The rotation of the cycle defines a centre. That centre is you. In alchemy the changes were called *circulatio*, a continual cycling of primal matter or life-stuff, leading to a union of opposites. The opposites to be united are the two opposing excellences: ovulation and menstruation. If either does not engage its counterpart it becomes isolated and troubled. The dark side, whichever side it is for the individual, is explored through the mandala and brought into the light, so it knows and likes itself. Then it grows to know and like its sister culmination, and the two unite into an awareness of the whole cycle. 'One does not become enlightened by imagining figures of light, but by making the darkness conscious.'[3]

Using the menstrual mandala one can discover a great variety of events that would otherwise remain unnoticed. If there are negative symptoms which recur, these will be clear. Knowing *when* will help towards *why*. Tuning in to enjoyable or creative moments will also render these more visible and so more *reliable*, and noticing them will very likely increase their frequency. It is only recently that psychologists have been noticing positive events. Lo and behold, they discover that something like 20 per cent of women find their premenstrual week full of positive energies – so it's not all PMS! Remember, dreaming will be found to take the place of unpleasant symptoms: when there is active vivid dreaming, then PMS is at a minimum.

Many will find links with the moon, tides and the weather, and many too a hitherto unconscious rhythmic link with a male partner or their children, through dreaming, or shared symptoms, or creative times. More than one woman has noticed that during her period her children are most busy at making things for themselves or each other. One male artist puts it this way: 'When my partner's period comes it usually marks the resolution of some creative struggle. It is as though a benign presence had entered the house, and, like the blood, my work flows satisfactorily.'

It is best not to use just a diary for recording symptoms or other events. A page a week just won't show anything at a glance. Of course, a written journal is needed to record dreams in detail, but it needs to be coded to a diagram that shows the movement of forces and events instantly.

The most important thing is to know your pattern. Knowing your cycle can shrink the difficult times. If they arrive unexpectedly, they can have a domino effect, upsetting more than the days they belong to. This is why our advice is to insert on the mandala or any kind of chart the *good* times as well. Not to do this is like making a map of the countryside, putting in all the quicksands and graveyards and quite omitting 'areas of outstanding natural beauty'.

It is important to realize that women can be persuaded into expecting the cycle to be bad at the usual pre-menstrual time. This then becomes a self-fulfilling prophecy, as the cycle, like the human imagination, is very sensitive to suggestion: 'I should feel bad; I'll look; yes, I do.' What is being registered here may be a passing perception, such as reaction to the weather. With the mandala an event like this may very well become integrated into the larger pattern.

Using the menstrual mandala you can see when the lows and highs happen; men making a similar chart may find that they have as many or more episodes of depression than women. The cycle can be a strong and organizing structure because from it you learn your interior rhythm. Moreover, you can look for the reasons behind any difficult variation.

For example, a woman who has decided to have no more children may suffer PMS in the whole last fortnight of the cycle, from just before ovulation onwards. Yet it is quite likely that the really sensitive time is the transition to ovulation. It is sensitive because it is now a non-eventful section of her cycle, which she has, so to speak, given up. She is really travelling hopefully to meet the menstrual experience, instead of the ovulation one, so anything on the way is full of repressed energies. The dreams will show this, enabling her to respond with understanding. A good transition-dream will ease her over the mid-cycle scratchiness. Now she does not miss the point of insight at which she could resolve; and instead of fourteen days of inappropriate PMS, accepts some passing scratchiness on just those sensitive days.

The mandala can be kept at a simple level, or it can be elaborated according to taste. The larger pattern, of a season or year, will show up by comparing monthly charts. Looking back over a year or more one can see how the period's length and timing may alter according to the seasons, the weather, the rise and fall of symptoms, of sexuality, of children's or partner's illnesses and joys. The year thus acquires a physical shape, and one can see how one month affects another.

Womanly insight and ingenuity will devise forms of self-representation and environmental responses that nobody now can guess at! An artist could make of her months a winding conch big enough to enter, and contemplate from within, or a great worm, segmented with the moon; an artist-scientist could find unguessed-of rhythms and patterns between inner and outer and maybe discover the operation of senses hitherto neglected; a musician could turn it to sound, its complex harmonics to music. People of an astronomical bent will be able to make moon-calendars with the moon-phase for each of the 365 days shown, and mark a lot of information in its spaces. This clearly is for people who feel the importance of the moon, and is an act of attention to that strong environmental rhythm.

The shape of our simple mandala is like that of the spider-web, beloved by the Greenham Common women. Ancient tradition might name it Arionrhod's Wheel, the Ferris of Fairies' Wheel, the Philosopher's Wheel, the Wheel of Fortune and Love. We hope one day to unite the old and the new by commissioning software for the menstrual mandala. Then it will be easy to find and visualize the many patterns that the balancing forces of the cycle must make within itself, and in response to the world.

5. Dream-rhythms

Dreaming is rhythmical. Every night we sink down into the depths of dreamless sleep, but, like Alice in her Wonderland rabbit-hole, as we go down we dream; but we also dream as we ascend. There are many episodes of dreaming each night, and we can elect to recall a good deal more of this dreaming than we commonly allow. The clue is to *believe*. The dream-agent is rather like a child of genius, sulking in a corner. She is sulking because we refuse to take any notice of her. She is a genius of creativity, but, in most of us, she is still a child, and can be coaxed out only when we show her that we believe that dreams are important. We must help the dream-agent to come out of her menstrual seclusion.

An earnest interest will always give access to dreams. You have to say, however inconvenient, 'I will record this dream'. That bargain struck, the dream will come. Put the date at the head of your notes, as well as the day of the cycle. And mark 'dream' on the mandala. It is best always to have paper and pencil by the bed. You may wake and mull over the dream before moving, carefully and gently, to set it down. Perhaps you will make rapid notes, and fill them in later. It is important to move gently, as you can either wake too far too soon, or the very movement in the half-sleeping state may give rise to other dreams, half-dreams and secondary revisions. It is important to note the 'mere fragments' – often these are aphoristic and full of meaning. A small tape-recorder is handy.

People say, 'Oh, I never dream', but everybody does. One reason for not recalling them is the unfamiliarity of the images. Reading a book about dreams actually helps you to dream. The dreams recorded in this book will have a similar effect. Life-questions are engaged, and a vocabulary of images is provided which a sincere resolve can turn into progressive stories on subsequent nights. Often a big dream comes on the first night of real dreaming, and may unravel in several chapters in subsequent dreams.

A frequent beginning-dream is of a good deal of coming and going in trains and stations. This can be a kind of tuning to the timetables of the cycle. Initially too there may be many car dreams: the brakes have gone, the car is lost. It is quite important in the dream-quest to lose the car. A car is usually a false face, and a symbol of the outer consumerist world. It is an unhealthy pram, an insulating infantilism, an armouring.

On freer mobilization of one's dream-psyche there may be dreams of many people aimlessly moving about. These people then start moving in patterns, sitting down at meals, or pacing in circles. If they do the last they are defining a centre, and the next step is to see what is in the centre. Seeing this, whatever it is, can then open a new dream-series.

Images may be strongly synaesthetic – that is, one may taste a visual impression or smell a colour, especially pre-menstrually or menstrually. This and other dream-events can be confusing but practice will allow the dream to stretch out, as it were, and become easier. Often the urgency of a neglected truth will distort a dream with its emphasis, as a voice is distorted by anger. One's children's dreams often show a simpler version of one's own, including cycle imagery.

Nightmares are very important, and are treasures. They are terrifying because something one doesn't wish to know has been repressed and is now forcing itself, in a concentrated form, into your attention.

One woman dreamed that she got out of bed because she heard somebody thumping at the front door. She went down and opened it, and saw nothing there. Then she looked down and saw something waiting on the threshold like an enormous ridged and fluted molar the size of a big typewriter. As she watched, it began to bounce up and down, until it was bouncing as high as her knees with a kind of rubbery sentience. She stood aside to let it pass, and it bounced up the stairs and paused at the first bedroom, which was the dreamer's. Then it started bouncing again, bounced into the children's bedroom and stopped at the elder child's bed, bouncing higher as if to get a look at the sleeping face. Then the bounces took the great tooth over to the younger boy's bedside and it bounced here too, higher and higher, so as to see the sleeping face, but this time it bounced sideways. It landed on the face and by squeezing its substance crushed it so that blood spurted across the white pillow.

The dreamer woke screaming. Her male partner comforted her. In the morning her period had come, and she was calmer, but it was clear that the nightmare had deeply shocked her. As she was a sculptor her partner suggested that she model the tooth in order to exorcise its form, but she refused. She had not worked in a long time, and was going through a sterile patch.

The man had to go away for a while, and when he came back he found that she had modelled the tooth in terra-cotta. It was a fearsome object, like the biggest tooth of the greatest dinosaur, all fluted at the sides and ridged over the upper grinding surface. But round the big terra-cotta model were many smaller works, all figures, on the table, on the mantelpiece, on the floor.

'Where did these come from?' he asked. 'I thought you couldn't work!'

'I saw them in the flutings of the tooth,' she said. 'Look, you can see them there too. All I did was to model them from what I saw in it.'

This nightmare, actually composed of the compressed forms of work that had been unconsciously 'cooked' within, had pressed hard and invisibly on her during her long artistic sterility, and had pressed through in the form of a nightmare just before her period. It had ushered in a new creative time in which the forms unfolded like Japanese paper flowers in water. But there was more to it than this.

The first, smaller, figures that she had so prolifically modelled were striking. They were of a man and woman facing each other and fastened in that position by the kissing faces and the genitals. They had a dynamic quality as though they were at once pushing towards each other in the embrace, and at the same time pulling away, but unable to break free.

A second series showed a man and a woman facing away from each other, but still fastened together down the sides, like Siamese twins. During the weeks further series appeared to the artist's eye in the flutings and grinding surface. These included a very relaxed female figure lounging by itself on a couch, and a series of terra-cotta tiles which opened in the centre to vagina-like structures, open, unoccupied, free. It also became clear during those weeks that the sculptor's relationship to her male partner was now over. However, before the figures declared it, neither had had the courage to admit this.

This is strange, but stranger things happen in 'the glamour of upset', especially late during the pre-menstrual quadrant, the fourth week. If they do, it is important to admit them and 'as a stranger bid them welcome'. Whatever the mechanism by which this may be mediated, this time of the month *seeks blood*. Minor accidents will occur. Cut fingers are frequent. Sometimes this will bring the period on, as if the cycle has to be primed with preliminary blood. One boy developed a kind of varicose vein in his perineum during a distressed PM time of his mother. It bled slightly and his GP said he didn't know what it was. After the period it disappeared, and has not recurred.

A therapist engaged in daily dream analysis with a woman over some eight months bled from his anus on the morning of the day the period was due, on five consecutive months.

A seven-year-old lost a milk-tooth with a great deal of blood on each of her mother's five successive late pre-menstrual occasions. Another woman not only dreamed of her daughter as the powerful young witch, but the older woman's cycle began to synchronize with the daughter's, moving round until the two bled together, strongly.

Yet another woman had a boyfriend who regarded himself as a kind of god. It was as though he would not admit his mortality, he had such self-confidence. During one late pre-menstrual phase the woman had a small car accident that jolted her and started her period. Almost simultaneously the man sheared the top off one of his fingers at work. The astonishment of this 'synchronicity' altered the attitude of both radically. The bond deepened as both had shed blood at the same time – the man accepted his mortality and vulnerability as a fact of life.

There are sometimes events during this charged pre-menstrual time that almost deserve the label 'clairvoyance'. One woman believed that she had caused a fire at an art school by means of bad-wishing, a fire in which her errant boyfriend's portfolio was destroyed. She was greatly distressed by this, until she was convinced that she had merely predicted it, but there were certain details in her late pre-menstrual dream that were accurate and could not have been known to the dreamer beforehand. In this phase of the cycle ordeals by fire and witch-burnings are frequent dreams. The power of the pre-menstrual phase is sought in certain magical or Wiccan rites, under the patronage of the goddess Sekhmet, of whom more later.

ALCHEMY FOR WOMEN

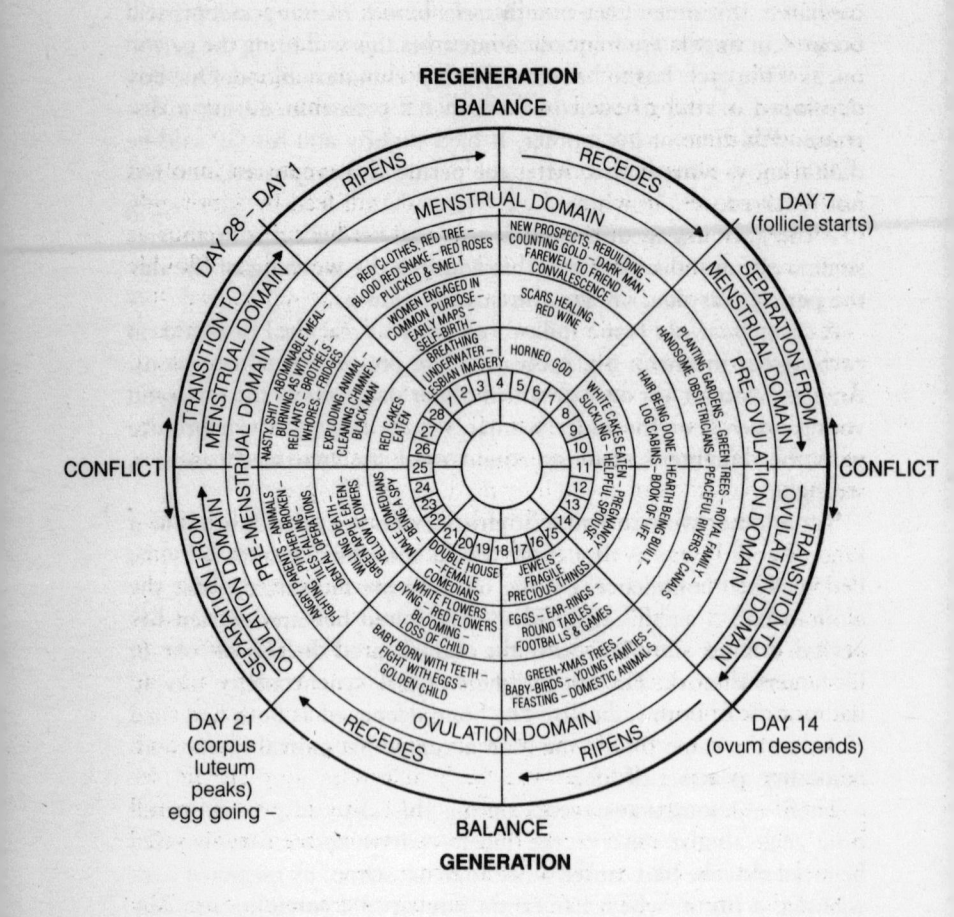

Figure 2. *The Mandala of the Menstrual Cycle*
Dreams tend to a characteristic imagery according to their position in the cycle. The figure shows approximate cycle locations of some frequent images in several womens' dreams.

Using the mandala is like using a weather-map: it teaches one to notice with one's feelings the signs of approaching changes or existent happenings, it is a tuning-device and a learning-process, a compass to the magnetic fields of the great images. So with dreams: using the mandala stimulates them and arouses the collective vocabulary within which the individual happenings play. Dreaming is strengthened by knowing the rhythms, as this is a going-with them.

Sharing dreams with other people will also create an involved feed-back process in which the told dream will feed back not only to the consciousness of the partner, but to her/his subconscious as well, creating more dreams. This is a process we call the 'double pelican', after the alchemical instrument of that name, and this constant circular distillation of images and feelings produces a new spirit of sharing, since the conscious of one person reacts to the unconscious of the other. One warning: share dreams only with partners or close friends. If you tell them too often to strangers the dream-agent quickly becomes insulted, as dreams are meant to be *felt*. (For more information, see Chapter 15.)

If you are really committed and the dream-agent is convinced that you are interested, there will be no shortage of dreams. People who 'never dream' may have to start off by setting the alarm clock for half-past three in the morning, which nearly always catches a good dream, but one probably won't have to do this more than once or twice before regular dreaming starts up without the stimulus.

A good way of stimulating a dream or waking dream is to do a relaxation practice. You can use the Eeman relaxation circuit (see pages 85–6), or the reverie after sex, and gently request with full belief: 'Please give me a dream that shows me my menstrual cycle.' You should not have to do this more than once.

Sealed writing (see pages 144–5) stimulates dreaming, especially when the packet is opened and read after at least a month. Sealed writing is a form of controlled waking dreaming. Dreams recorded over the month will chime with and develop the waking entries, creating another 'double pelican' situation as dream-self and waking-self move towards each other.

Dream-creatures and persons are living things, and should be treated as creatures in their own right. One must try to feel into their lives – especially the lives of the ones that seem monstrous.

They are not there to illustrate or allegorize the menstrual cycle: the menstrual cycle is their means of contact. The cycle is a powerful instrument of communication, but what speaks through it is not just 'egg' or 'blood' but one's deep self which, after all, came from egg through birth-blood. That self naturally may have important things to say about 'egg' and 'blood', but they are not 'nothing but' egg and blood. The cycle gives access to these messengers who appear as if through revolving doors. The pattern is a natural one, like any body pattern, such as the circulatory rhythm, and is in that sense an eternal pattern. But the energy known as 'egg' or 'blood' is not to be explained away or dismissed by saying 'It's just the cycle'. It is more that these messages extend the meanings of 'egg' and 'blood' so that one sees at the same time that such eternal, archetypal images are also intimately one's own. The proper attitude is one of amazement that these things hold such meaning, when before they were dismissed.

Active, creative work can take some of the dream-time from the night, and so substitute for it that one does not necessarily dream as much as usual. People not accessing dreams should try nutritional remedies if there is no medical objection – men too! We mentioned above that a 'smelling' dream shows the conscious passing of a difficult threshold; conversely, the practice of aromatherapy will stimulate dreaming and give imagery that assists its passage.

Beginning homoeopathic treatment often starts an important dream-series. Homoeopathy appears to stimulate the immune system, and dreams may be partly a kind of consciousness of the immune system. The mandala will show that sex and a recalled dream often go hand in hand.

Taking on such inward-feeling practices as inspecting the cervix and the mucus will stimulate dreaming as well, and reduce premenstrual trouble; as with the dream-agent, the cycle responds to sincere interest. Even when the cycle has been neglected for a long time, it is not too late. Feeling the softness and movement of the cervix must be one of the most ancient forms of guided imagining and feeling-within. Sometimes women are given in a dream the images of a quiet place or beautiful solitude, and they can use this in imagination and thereby deepen a relaxation. Sometimes there is a spontaneous vision, a place with a navel-stone, or it may be a small grassy hillock, like the cervix, among trees. Deep feelings can come from inspecting tenderly the entrance to the womb, the birth-cone, called by the ancients Omphalos, the centre of life, where two worlds meet.

6. Some Warnings and Encouragements

A centrally important symbol encountered in the dreams is that of the animus, the image of the male side of the female psyche. Its appearance can reflect a personal problem with men or a more general, cultural, one with masculinity. His dream anger may coincide with the pre-menstrual syndrome, but the principle holds that if he is dreamed, then there is less physical suffering.

To acknowledge the animus is certainly not to say that a woman is really a man within, or anything like it. This would be a profound misunderstanding. It is best to say that the animus of the woman may symbolize the relationship between herself and her unconscious mind, the unknown countries within. There are other figures, both male and female, who may do this, but that known as the animus is usually the most active and transforming.

If there has been or is conflict with the father, for example, and if the father has a problem in his attitude to women, then there will be an angry or cold animus in the dreams, often appearing at the end of the third week (ovulation separation). Masculine education wishes to allow little power to women except as mothers, and it has been shown statistically that the daughters of college-educated fathers are more likely to suffer paramenstrual distress than if the father does not have that background. Similarly, it has been found that paramenstrual distress is more likely in orthodox Jewish families where the blood is regarded as unclean, and in Catholic families, where the woman as mother is exalted, than in Protestant families.[1]

The animus as a dream-figure will have a different character according to whether he represents the ovulation or the menstruation side of the cycle. It is the menstrual animus who commonly gives the most frights and the best rewards. As he represents menstrual powers, he is the witchmaster. He appears post-ovulation as the dark sinister figure, as a vampire, as a strange man of unknown powers, the other husband. An animal may accompany him, or he may appear himself as a power-animal. He may appear as an assembly of animals of archaic form, termites or ants, for instance; here the problem is that he cannot be conversed with in this form, so communication (or the clear transfer of energy) cannot occur on the conscious level. He is frequently fragmented into multitudes and may appear as an army of privates (the dream would intend a pun) or the Houses of Parliament; if the latter, one needs the Speaker – the message must be integrated into a helpful form rather than all the Members shouting at once.

Animus may appear as a bright angel of ovulation, as to the Virgin Mary. He can also be a dark angel, or an angel falling in flames. This image of falling Lucifer with flaming hair is quite frequent, and depicts the hot energies of the menstruating womb (the 'demon's head') and the fall from the 'heaven' of child-bearing and ovulation. So it will seem to some quite a wicked image to dream, and this is how guilt arises. When such a dream is resisted, it turns into physical distress. Knowledge of what the dream is saying relieves the pain and guilt. Equally, the menstrual animus may appear as the Horned God of the Witches, and this is a reflection of the womb as the demon's head, with its 'horns' of the Fallopian tubes, ready to impart menstrual 'magic'.

The menstrual animus may appear as a child, but specifically *the child you never had*. It is as if when the egg is not fertilized, it gives up its energies to form a dream-child who can communicate with its mother-who-is-no-mother. Recognition of this very helpful figure, who can burst through with extreme menstrual distress (which subsides as he is recognized), was probably once an accepted magical or psychological technique. There are ancient Egyptian documents which are a kind of sung counterpoint between Isis and her dark sister Nephthys of the underworld, the Egyptian Persephone, representing menstrual energies. The song or litany is an appeal to the spirit of the man-child either to incarnate or to give counsel as a spirit. Sometimes the goddess Isis is depicted with her earrings in the form of the Tet-buckle (a design like a little red human figure signifying Isis' redeeming blood) as though she were menstruating, and listening to this counsellor.

It is sometimes said that witches would deliberately miscarry, coat the foetus in pitch, a 'tar baby', and hang the effigy on a tree.[2]

The spirit of the child would perch like a bird in this tree, and give counsel. Menstrual cloths might be used instead, and this is probably the origin of the 'wishing tree' of Japan and Cornwall to which one ties cloths, which are wishes, which come true as the cloths disintegrate in the weather.

A tree is itself a very powerful machine of electricity and perfume, and we can learn to respond to it as a waking gateway to dream-life by placing our own energies in its fields. A walk among trees can be like a waking dream relieving the electrical tension of PMS or POS; one should lay one's back against its trunk and feel the life-currents flowing.

The ovulation animus, on the other hand, is the inner image of everything which promotes home and family and the rearing of children. He is kind and supportive, often a professional man, a doctor or musician, a man-figure who might easily find his way into the motor-car advertisements or the Sunday colour supplements or a musical comedy. But one has to be exceedingly careful of him: there are certain matters one cannot mention in his presence, at the risk of his explosive anger. His politics are right-wing and he dislikes anything that is 'not like us'. His brightness casts a very dark shadow (in the form of his intimate antagonist, the menstrual animus) because to him menstruation is murder and witchcraft, and in him is the puritan who loves to burn witches. Superman, whose shoulders are broad and whose sex is rudimentary, is a clean-cut avatar of the ovulation animus, while the Phantom of the Opera presides over the mysteries of inspiration of the menstrual period. The Phantom of the Opera is a mutilated personage who inspires a singer and teaches her music in the cellars of the opera house, who hides his bleeding wound, who has been unjustly exiled by the machinations of ovulation figures piling up money for their future dynasties, and who appears at the masked ball as skull-faced death, robbed in opulent scarlet. The libretto of the popular musical has him sing that he 'Wallows in blood yet denies love'! This haunting story is itself a significant pattern of feminine dreaming.

It must be remembered that any man or woman can become 'possessed' by such unconscious figures, and behave as stereotypes. Ulanov gives an eloquent example of this, when a woman's ego is partially identified with her animus:

[A] primitive, unconscious power drive, a ruthless egotism

masked by outward compliance or helplessness. She seems an interested listener but she hears nothing but a confirmation of her own opinions. She seems compassionate but she insists relentlessly on getting her own way. She forces her help on another to ensure that it is clear that she is needed. She is the one who seems to be trying to understand, but in fact she persistently misconstrues meanings and insinuates opposing purposes into conversations.[3]

This 'possession' can be temporary, and pre-menstrual, as the forceful animus energies rise up with the cycle. If it goes with a dream, the dreamer may now 'possess' this figure. Many professional women, understanding the force of this animus, may deliberately call on this pre-menstrual force and use its patterns to master conflict at other times of the cycle. Thus its power must not be underestimated, nor its value. Because men are seen as behaving in this fashion, her unconscious perceives the source of the pattern, she heals herself and comes into her power. But power is not the only thing to live by.

Thus the alternative to this or another such unconscious possession is to possess the figure oneself, and this can be done by relating to its symbolized qualities in a dream. Dreaming and taking consistent note of dreams as they appear and reappear in the cycle is the way to self-possession. Recurrent dreams are very important, and often recur in relation to some particular cycle-stage. To understand this is to stop the dreams recurring; they will move on and develop in other ways.

The weight-gain and depression, the hydration, craving for sweets, breast-tenderness and other symptoms of separation PMS can be looked upon as possession by the ovulation spirit, and an unwillingness both mental and physical to let go of the possibility of having a child as the menstrual events come nearer. Animus-anger, his craving to be a child, his breast-feeding denied him, emerges as symptoms, or dreams.

On the other hand, one can see in, say, transition PMS, the mood swings, irritability, forgetfulness, confusion and all such mental intrusions of that witch Phantom, the inspired singing-teacher of menstruation, whose gifts of a life alternative to possession by the family and children are beginning to be unlocked by women. Of course his raucous knocking on the mirror-door, his crude phantasmagoria, are a result of his long exile; even his gender identifies the source of the problem: the Oedipal society which denies women the symmetry of their rhythms. Indeed, the Oedipus complex is the form the ovulation instinct takes in men: they marry mothers.

Any of these problems may be experienced in the PMS or POS couvade: this is the upset the man may undergo in synchronization with the woman's cycle (see Chapter 7). This is equivalent to the better known couvade at child-bearing, when the man suffers real or imagined labour pains. So much PMS originates from the man's difficulty – both psychological and physiological – in passing with ease through the threshold changes in harmony with the woman's.

To put the whole matter another way: those women who are attuned to the conventional female values of the mother and the home are disappointed by the approach of the period, and tend to suffer from the hydration and craving forms of PMS; while those women of a more exploratory and magical cast of mind – artists, poets, what the psychologists call 'divergers' – can suffer both from the separation PMS which is the repressed energy of ovulation separation, if it is not resolved, and also from the transition PMS which is withheld knowledge of the pre-menstrual crossing, the approaching period. Not recognizing the imminence of this crossing could lead to a possession as severe as the disappointed pregnancy in the converger, possibly of waywardly sexual and 'whorish' or 'witchy' behaviour. Disappointed of pregnancy, the practised woman dreamer awaits her consultation with the spirit of the child which was not to be, in its many mercurial disguises.

By careful use of the menstrual mandala, we can actually possess information about when and how and in what pattern these events occur; and we are not continually recovering from overwhelming physical troubles associated with the cycle. We can do this too by meeting in groups and comparing experiences; taking care that the groups are well balanced so that women whose interest is motherhood do not cast women whose interests lie elsewhere in the role of witchy shadows; nor the reverse, mothers seen as stodgy instead of the channel of the generations, while the 'witches' are the discoverers and scientists of a new world of feeling and vision.

Chief, then, among the recurrent images are those that depict the man-problem in a woman, and the woman-problem in a man. To state the dilemma another way: when we are children we are not neuter, but rather deuter, composed of the two genders. When puberty arrives, one of these genders goes underground and becomes unconscious, consciousness being taken up with the induction into the given gender role, depending on the customs of the society.

This does not mean that the opposite gender in a person disappears. Far from it. It is now partly unconscious, and therefore acts as a messenger and a catalyst from the unconscious.

In a man this figure is the anima. It is a living image of the man's woman-problem, which also carries and reserves the feminine power and knowledge. The man may very likely project his anima upon actual women, and in so far as he does so, he is relating to his own self, for good or ill. Kept unconscious, the anima makes a man subject to moody and even violent 'adolescent' behaviour, which may be cyclical and related to a partner's menstrual events. If, however, he meets the anima in her menstrual mutations, he may complete his partial nature by solving what for him was 'the woman-problem'. He is no longer possessed by her but develops and possesses those qualities which society reserves as more proper to a woman, as a part of his own character.

The woman's psyche is parallel in this. Her man-image, and with it all the man-problems of otherness and unrelatedness, will be formed on a basis provided by her father and brothers and early experiences, which can of course include sexual abuse. Thus she takes in the man-problem through her pores throughout her life. At times of stress, images symbolizing this unsolved man-problem will come up. The unconscious animus, as we have pointed out, may possess her; typically she behaves like a bossy, argumentative and immature man, very opinionated. But if she encounters the animus figure in her dreams or waking dreams, then she is able to relate to him as a woman rather than be possessed by him. He will be the repository of qualities which have been reserved by society as more proper to the man, and therefore denied to her in so far as she is a woman, and relating to him will help her recover these for her own use.

But it is as though each animus has two levels. The first is that the archetype (the basic great symbol) carries all the qualities and deficiencies of patriarchal society and its values too. It is possible that if women were brought up in a society in which none of the values was represented by men, they would carry no animus, any more than they would carry left-brain lateralization (indeed, the two may be the same thing). But as it is, to become whole, a woman must deal with the image of the male that has been branded in her mind from her earliest contacts with men, through her education, largely man-centred, to her marriage and beyond. In particular, the animus becomes shadowed by man's menstrual neglect, so when culminations of the cycle arrive, this figure is very active – taking on the guise of the damager to draw attention to the nature of the damage.

Another level of the animus is sheer animal and sheer spirit. He is not only the human animal, but the Other who is animal too, and by a curious paradox of the unconscious thereby as much spirit as animal. As animal he can be a male Sphinx; as spirit, Lord of the Underworld kidnapping and raping Persephone, sheer earth-power.

The animality can be archaic and diffuse, can be imaged as we instanced at the period in the form of a swarm of red ants. A dream-series during the paramenstruum may condense diffused or swarming animals like these into creatures with whom it is easier to relate: in succession a talking snake, sometimes crowned; or warm-blooded animals like cats or dogs; nearly-human like monkeys. The animal images are there to restore right-brain values and the dark senses that are non-visual and which the animals share in a world more full of relatedness and inter-communication than we can easily imagine. They are the animals of Eden.

The dream cycle once grasped is direct inner knowledge independent of masculine tradition. In fact, much masculine tradition may be founded in unconscious recognition of the stages of the cycle. Sir James Frazer's famous and influential exploration of mythologies, *The Golden Bough*, sets out as its main theme to solve the mystery of the savage cult of the priest-kings of Diana's sanctuary at Nemi.

> In this sacred grove there grew a certain tree round which at any time of the day, and probably far into the night, a grim figure might be seen to prowl. In his hand he carried a drawn sword, and he kept peering warily about him as if at every instant he expected to be set upon by an enemy. He was a priest and a murderer; and the man for whom he looked was sooner or later to murder him and hold the priesthood in his stead.[4]

This famous passage, which initiates Frazer's quest through thirteen large volumes, could equally well be the pre-menstrual dream of a modern woman. The cycle itself is often symbolized in dreams as the Tree of Knowledge and of Life, on which moon-fruits ripen. The two murderous tanists, successive priest-kings, symbolize the dual male guardianship of the feminine, and the killing the transition from one state to the other, ineluctably repeated. They were supposed to guard the mistletoe, the golden bough that is the light in the underworld, and this would symbolize dream knowledge.

The menstrual mandala itself looks like a slice of that tree, and many such cycles build up its trunk. The Cross of Jesus is said to be made from the wood of the Tree of Life in the garden of Eden. What we see in the menstrual mandala is the feminine cross, on which the woman is crucified by the crossing or crux of those alternative modes, ovulation and menstruation. From one state she dies to the other, and visits the underworld of hell of that unknown state, and her harrowing of hell is the release of the pagan dead, of the repressed material of history, or 'herstory'. Knowing the lost world, she returns, resurrected, with the treasures of the underworld in her arms. Perhaps the myth of Jesus owes its importance and power to the symbolic suggestion that the male is here prepared to follow the immemorial pattern of the willing sacrifice and the Crossing. It is in that case surprising that women priests have never been appointed to be the leaders in this mystery in 2,000 years, though they may have established it. This would explain why a man should dream pre-menstrually of a crucified woman.

Popular entertainments of very wide appeal may reflect the cycle patterns, like collective waking dreams. Indeed, they would not be popular if they did not. Most musicals are largely on the ovulation side, like *Seven Brides for Seven Brothers*, seven days of the ovulation quadrant. Some, equally popular, can show the whole pattern with ovulation animus and menstrual animus embattled for the soul of the woman. *King Kong* has the gigantic ape fighting for the heroine against the human hero. The ape dies in New York among the sky-scrapers of ovulatory, consumerist America which wishes to treat Kong as no more than an entertainment, until he breaks loose and is shot down.

As mentioned above, *The Phantom of the Opera* is an excellent example. The plot hinges on whether the gifted female singer will marry a titled man and breed his dynasty, or whether she will follow her art and become a great singer. She is inspired to sing by the

Phantom, the 'Angel of Music', a murderous figure of great mystery haunting the immense behind-the-scenes of the Paris Opera, who masks half his face, who dresses as Death in scarlet, whose loving emblem is a red rose, and who opens a passage through mirrors to the life of inspired music. He is a perfect dream-figure of the menstrual animus. *The Phantom of the Opera* is like a collective waking dream of menstrual initiation.

Dr Jekyll and Mr Hyde is another popular myth that shows the splitting of the personality into the two forms of animus: this splitting may often occur in the dreams of both men and women and in a man's conduct. The story originally came to R. L. Stevenson as a dream. In a dream-series, though, there are four appearances possible to this kind of man figure. At ovulation he might be benevolent Dr Jekyll but, if the egg is not fertilized, benevolent Dr Jekyll may very well become worried, angry Dr Jekyll who drinks his potion and is transformed to malevolent Hyde, who then changes to benevolent Hyde as the period and its mysteries near. In the films, Spencer Tracy's Hyde was simply Jekyll with more energy and different eyebrows; director Rouben Mamoulian turned Fredric March into an authentic Neanderthal man who loves the smell of the air and the rainfall, but who is as patriarchal in his attitudes as Jekyll, and differs only in enacting them murderously. The film has yet to be made in which the smooth doctor mutates into an energetic doctor who acts militantly on behalf of the prostitutes instead of murdering them. Jekyll's potion in a dream would represent menstrual blood, drunk in a ritual manner to enhance its effects. Tracy's Jekyll dreams the pollution of a woman's body by a great muddy dinosaur claw, the archaic approach of the period interpreted by post-ovulation attitudes.

The immensely popular *Nightmare on Elm Street* series of films feature an energetically destructive and fiery menstrual animus called affectionately 'Freddie' – the physically solid, apparently flayed and fire-coloured avatar or resurrected bodily form of a child-murderer who was burnt to death by outraged parents. This sardonic, wise-cracking entity has the power to steal the souls of children by encountering and killing them in their dreams. He can be temporarily destroyed, but pops up again apparently at will. In the last film of the series he is dissolved by being forced to see his own reflection within the dream. The souls he has captured stream out of him up to heaven, the individual complexes or souls which comprised him are liberated. The cycle turns again and the young people are free to resume their mating rituals – until Freddie returns. But he is still the dream-master whom everybody loves to hate, and who raises creative powers and promotes self-realization in those powerful enough to outface him by their endurance and ingenuity. *Nightmare on Elm Street* is another parable of how urgent it is to encounter energies which are ugly from repression.

Perhaps the great popularity of stand-up 'alternative' comedians lies in the way in which they make their presence felt as a beneficent transforming animus in many women's dreams, a kind of benevolent Mr Hyde. They are people who get behind the scenes, know something is wrong, and have found a humorous pattering improvisatory right-brain style to embody their life-version and their protest. They seem to be masters of both worlds. This makes them good role-models on the menstrual side of a positive animus who keeps the dreamer conscious through the passage of difficult thresholds. Animal vitality and spirit combine, and if they are outrageously sexual, so be it. They raise power by their humour; with gusts of energy they transform a bad social situation where change seemed impossible to one in which solutions suddenly appear without warning. They unite an audience with their mercurial wit. Of course the menstrual animus is a rascal! What else could he be – killing a woman's baby and making her feel sexual about the killing – except a kind of divinity, knowing and practising such paradoxes of death into life and life into death as a Trickster! Negative emotions now seem generously funny; we are all human after all!

Comics such as Robin Williams, Ben Elton and Lenny Henry appear in women's dreams and function in this way; Elton has a particular concern with the environment, and he makes robust wholesome jokes about male menstruation – in one a famous cricketer 'comes on' as he is about to go in and bat. In another show he joked about men drinking together who suddenly had their periods in sympathy, like they always did, but because the Tampax-machine in the Gents was empty, they had to go home with beer-mats clasped between their legs.

Female comedians, like Dawn French, also appear as helpful same-sex companions; a comic action means a change of attitude in an impossible situation. One woman was held up in a dream by a precipitous cliff. Dawn French appeared and, making a joke,

THE INNER MEANING OF THE MOON CYCLE

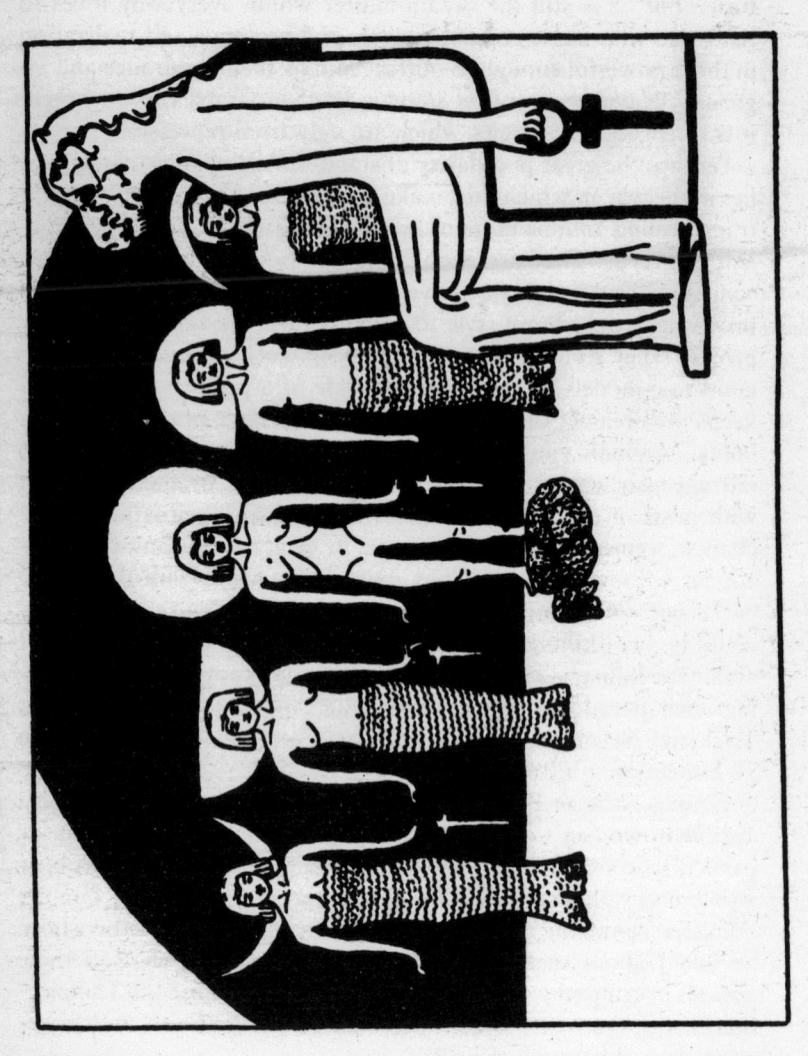

Figure 3. *Sekhmet and Moon Dream-Cycle*
From *Woman's Mysteries* by M. Esther Harding (1976)

stepped off the precipice. The air in her skirt buoyed her up, and she fluttered down, twirling with a circular motion which reminded the dreamer of the turning cycle itself, and of the sycamore key which resembles the clitoris, the tree of 'be sick no more'.

Sometimes the whole cycle appears in a dream in one stunning image and this image turns out to be a collective one, known from centuries before. There is a famous triad by an ancient Welsh poet, Peredur, Son of Efrawg: a poem which simply depicts a mystery:

> A tall tree on the river's bank,
> one half burning from root to top,
> the other half of it in green leaf.

More than one dreamer has seen this menstruation–ovulation tree in her dreams without knowing the Welsh poem, and when it has been pointed out to her she has gained a new respect for the dreaming process which can reach so far back in time.

There is a wonderful picture of the whole cycle in Esther Harding's important book *Woman's Mysteries*. It is the dream of a modern woman who saw a stage-set called 'The Phases of the Moon' or 'The Phases of the Goddess'. Against this set an individual drama composed of outer happenings – 'birth, marriage, death, work and social relationships' – is to be performed on the front of the stage.

The stage background, by contrast, represents 'on a deeper psychological level, the drama of the gods. This dream, since the dreamer was a woman, was represented by the phases of the Moon.' Five human figures are shown, each clasping a looped Egyptian cross, and bearing behind her head, respectively from left to right, a crescent moon, a waxing half-moon, a full moon, a waning half-moon, and a decrescent moon. Each figure has a fish-skin dress, receding down the body until at the middle full moon figure it lies discarded, touching her feet. The subsequent two figures resume the dress until the last is fully clothed. The features of the figures grow older, young at new moon, old at old moon. In the right foreground is a lion-headed goddess enthroned, holding a dark looped cross.

Esther Harding sees the fish-skin dress as unconscious instinct, which is fully discarded only at full moon (the traditional representation of ovulation); the opposite figure is a kind of 'mermaid or fish inhabiting the unconscious'. Harding comments:

> But this phase is not shown, for this phase of the woman is taboo; it is non-human, daemonic; it may not be spoken of, nor may it live in the light of day. It belongs to the sphere of the woman's mysteries. For a man to look on a woman then is 'sickness and death'.

This picture is somebody's menstrual mandala, showing the deep collective pattern against which the individual drama is composed, but at first sight it is a pattern that favours ovulation, as why should it not, in any individual. However, the dreamer might have liked to investigate what was being concealed from her use by that 'taboo'. The image of Sekhmet, an Egyptian sun-goddess, has been adopted by some modern feminist Wiccans to represent the solar energy and strength of the paramenstruum. Traditionally, this coincides with the dark moon, when it rises with the sun, and the power and energy of the preliminary pre-menstrual phase comes into play too. It may well be that this particular cycle-pattern shows the Motherhood cycle, with ovulation on the full moon – the figure of the Goddess is then representative of the energy of the unfertilized ovum, tabooed, but ready for the woman's use as it breaks up. Then the lioness rages because she is separated from her young; in the dream-picture her muzzle seems tearful.

However, some women have found that there is another cycle that coincides with the moon-phases, with menstruation on the full moon instead, and it is during this menstruation that they become 'fully human' with 'right-brain' activities. One may read the picture in either sense. Sekhmet could equally represent the goddess of ovulation; indeed, sunlight and golden suns are dream-images at ovulation, and the Goddess fierce for her offspring, and magnificent with her procreative power.

Some women find that if they do synchronize with the moon, as many women living out of cities do, that in maternal situations like school holidays, their period moves round so that menstruation comes at the dark moon; while during the school term or in non-maternal situations, menstruation tends to come on full moon. We call this alternative cycle the 'Wisewoman Cycle'. The Harding commentary says again that to ovulation menstruation is taboo, and vice versa. Sekhmet was an angry goddess, appeased by blood or beer. Her figure and attributes would therefore assist transitions in the cycle, blood of the approaching period, and beer for the festive atmosphere of traditional ovulation.

The picture is also making a comment about the looped cross, a popular contemporary ornament of great antiquity, the cross of life of the Egyptians. It is another form of the cross and circle, like the menstrual mandala. Perhaps we may see why it has its reputation. The human figures in this picture are evidently steering their way through transformations with this 'key of life'; it is as though the loop represents the vagina and the crossing into the vagina. The crux ansata (literally: cross with a handle) or ankh is held to represent the genitals of the Goddess Isis, the supreme goddess of life and death. Perhaps it shows more, with the head representing the crown of the clitoris, the cross-pieces the legs (or crura), and the vertical piece the vulva. It is an indubitable fact that self-stimulation to orgasm is a great and good way, as sex with a partner is, of disassembling oneself, as it were, and reconstituting on the other side of a threshold. It is thus the key to transformations.

Esther Harding's *Woman's Mysteries* is an important book that speaks out for the sacredness and power of menstruation, and the need for it to be an integral part of women's lives. She quotes a Vedic text: 'The blood of a woman is a form of Agni and therefore no one should despise it.' Agni is the fire-god. She says:

> In societies where the simple facts of nature are less controlled and distorted by personal or ego desires, the lives of women are arranged in a pattern dictated by their moon cycle. The social customs which prevail in so many parts of the world in relation to the woman's cycle were developed in part on account of man's fear of that in women which he did not understand. His fear doubtless contributed its share also to the development of the taboos controlling this aspect of feminine nature. For her sexual cycle had an uncanny power over him, arousing at once his own instinct and his dread of its power.[5]

We have seen how just and true these words are.

The crown and crura of the clitoris resemble exactly the maple or sycamore key, and this shape is a common dream-image for women. We attribute this to the fact that the dreamer in dreaming is always sexually excited. The male has an erection; the female becomes wet and the clitoris erects. This clitoris shape in dreams signifies, like the crux ansata, gentle, circular passage through the stages of the cycle, and the fluttering circular fall of the winged key reinforces this image through exterior observation (like Dawn French's fall earlier). Both sycamore and maple are famed as sacred trees, perhaps for this very good reason: the sycamore in Ancient Egypt, the maple in Amerindia. In Egypt the sycamore was sacred to the Black Goddess, the Goddess of Night, called Nuit, who was a patroness of the vision of the night, the dream.

It was one of the great achievements of the early contemporary women's movement to insist that there were times when self-stimulation to orgasm was entirely preferable to any partner at all; and that everybody, men included, should reserve that right. It may become particularly important in passing from late pre-menstrual to the menstrual stage, as there may be a sudden drop in ovarian hormones with the receding of the corpus luteum, and, in physiological terms, an orgasm can stimulate the womb's secretion of prostaglandins and neuro-transmitters. Cramps during the period and difficult flow are also helped by a self-induced orgasm and the reverie following that attends to the experience.

The inclination of our culture, which avoids the essential simplicities in case they give too much power to the individual, is to tell us that such matters as the interpretation of dreams are too difficult for the ordinary person, and that we need specialized dream analysts of various persuasions in a supervisory role. This is not the case, except in emergencies or when one is beginning one's approach to 'self-possession'. An experienced analyst, providing s/he does not avoid feminine knowledge, can 'mirror' the visions of the night and thus hold one's own imagery still enough for a time so that one can learn the language of one's own psyche. These explorations are so new (and yet so old) that once a woman dreamer lets go of her education and prejudices so much unfolds that it is beyond the experience of most men and most people of conventional training. It is the case that even the psychology of Jung, which is the closest yet devised to the feminine, conceals the basic patterns of feminine life. The rhythmic four-fold pattern which

SOME WARNINGS AND ENCOURAGEMENTS

Jung calls a mandala is indeed that magic circle we call the menstrual cycle, and Jungian alchemy is the male version of the correct self-management of that cycle. This is why men must work in all respects with their *Soror Alchymica*, 'Alchemical Sister'. Then wonders appear, mutual communications that are like thought transference, people dreaming each other's dreams in easier versions, menstrual distress lived out in an attenuated version by the men.[6]

Thus we find that once the basic work is done (that is, understanding the present form of one's period and the basic facts, so that some kind of menstrual mandala appears), then the dreams often explain themselves, and their energies lay themselves open to waking use. If we re-read our dream-journals after a lapse of time, with the patterned charts to hand, the knitting together of the dreams and the waking life becomes clear. Dreams may be shared both inside and outside the family, though only between people who are sincerely interested or willing to give it all a try.

The dreams declare themselves to the person who re-dreams in waking reverie and thought. Relaxation practice can enable one literally to re-dream them, or dream them further, as one takes the images and incidents down into the relaxation. So can telling one's dream in a group; one realizes suddenly that the dream is moving on a bit, and some room, some escarpment has shown itself which was concealed before. Sometimes the most useful dreams consist simply of a voice speaking a phrase.

All this happens if one can discern the underlying pattern to one's menstrual biorhythm. Once the woman is in possession of the basic facts, then the rest is common sense. This is why women, who have the rhythm in themselves, find dream-interpretation comes quite naturally, while in men it is so strenuous an activity. A woman experienced in dreams is not only grateful to Jung for emphasizing the four-fold patterns of the psyche, but she is also amused at his concealing it behind over-spiritualized imagery, hiding the fact that it is root-nature in the woman, from which the man learns. In Jungian doctrine it is the four functions that must be balanced in life: thought, feeling, sensation and intuition, and man does so by living their alternation through life. But it may be that women experience the revolution of these functions monthly and thus individuate no less than thirteen times a year (by menopause it is to be hoped that she has explored so far that she reaches a new totality). The so-called 'inferior function' is all important in Jungian psychology: this is the most energetic one that causes most trouble and needs most work, for integration. We have already seen that this function shows up plainly in the mandala, in one of the more difficult quadrants. Physical symptoms manifest themselves to begin with, then the more difficult dream imagery, reflecting realities in both worlds, the inner and the outer.

We mentioned in Chapter 1 that the first researchers in modern times ever to record women's dreams systematically in relation to the menstrual cycle were Therese Benedek and Boris Rubenstein. In 1942, they published discoveries of a vocabulary of dreams in the four phases. The cycle phase of the dream was confirmed by taking vaginal smears.

They found tense heterosexual dreams during the run-up to ovulation, that is, dreams involving the male figure we have called the 'ovulation animus'; relaxed and contented dreams associated with pregnancy and nursing in the ovulation and luteal phases; confused and energetic pre-menstrual dreams; and terrifying bloody dreams at menstruation itself. It is an indication of how matters have improved during the half-century since this work was published that, while Benedek and Rubenstein reported some vivid and fascinating menstrual dreams as 'regressive', women dreamers nowadays can see and respond more creatively to extraordinary menstrual dreams.

Here is one of their pre-ovulation dreams: 'Some huge fossil belonging to the reptile family, mounted, standing upright in the museum. Some remark or other brought it to life and it began to crawl over the land. People fled before it in terror. Very slimy and shining and ugly green.' Green is an ovulatory colour; the great prehistoric mother is being aroused.[7]

At ovulation: 'I asked the hostess if they had any eggs and she said they don't eat eggs in her home.' Naturally one doesn't eat eggs at ovulation, not in dreams anyway; however, the competitive mother-in-law ate eggs. Ovulation also is characterized by dreams of conflict with older women, or envy of other mothers. Witches – a menstrual power-image – are said to ride on broken eggshells.

Pre-menstruation can be the 'horror-film' time as the ovulation animus feels himself destroyed and becoming one of the 'living dead'. It is almost as if the rise of the cult of the horror-video has been a help to the dreamers of both sexes encountering the changes in the cycle, particularly the unexplored pre-menstrual and menstrual times. The murderous ovulation animus, baulked of physical life, may in dreams as well as films stagger about with decaying bits dropping off him. When this image is related to actual cycle happenings, however, its grip of fear goes, and the image can bid farewell, for the time being, sometimes in the image of a sailor-lover embarking on a voyage. This bitter-sweet image can replace earlier horrifying ones, and dreams of sailors in their 'berth' in the great belly of a ship are frequently symbolic of the 'little voyager', the unborn child.

The departing ovulation animus then gives way to the menstrual animus who, nourished by cultural fantasy in books and films, may reveal himself as the knowledgeable reborn magician or warlock whose blood-magic gives him power over animals, or he may himself be a were-animal with greatly enhanced sensory powers and consequent understanding. In his power he may seem the very devil, the horned man, the God of the Witches who, in tradition at least, has mastery of the menstrual powers. Courage in these dreams is often needed, as with Havelock Ellis's brave pre-menstrual dreamer, who said: 'I have to *decide* to walk through deep water, fully clothed. I have a fear of deep water.'[8]

The paradox of the fantasies of horror films is that one *enjoys* them, despite one's fright. Now that taboo material has become a familiar part of our world of fantasy, the images can begin to grow beyond fantasy-play to health, carrying with them their great energy, towards better imagination. Thus in one Benedek–Rubenstein dream there is a headless body, with a hideous bloody gash. The dreamer keeps repeating, 'It's all so hopeless', but then she deliberately goes over to the hideous corpse. 'Suddenly the girl was standing on the sidewalk. Her head was on her body again and she appeared to be more cheerful, as though she didn't fear that it would be detached again.' Something has given this woman confidence, so that she is no longer afraid of 'losing her head' at the bloody threshold. Indeed, the aim is to pass all the thresholds of the cycle without 'being possessed' but in full self-possession.

A practised dreamer will pass the thresholds of her cycle consciously, without a handicapping disruption of personality. Each cycle will bring new material into consciousness, new terrors and pleasures. So far, there do not appear to be many professional dream-analysts who bring this self-evident factor into their practice; we believe that without some approach to this cycle-knowledge, psychological work is derelict. However, there are many practised dreamers among women, and their numbers are increasing all the time, as the benefits and wonders of feminine dreaming grow more manifest and undeniable.

A man can also become a practised dreamer, and his dreams will show cyclical form if he is engaged seriously with a woman, and has studied the cycle, as the following account by a man acknowledges:

'A Vision at Tintagel. A tall part of the keep, the outer keep. Its foundations said to be older than the castle. Within sight of Merlin's cave? I meditated there by letting my roots down. Everything proceeded with a calm and lack of surprise, while the vision was actually occurring seen with an inner eye. I went down along the roots, through minerals, golden minerals and earth. Then I came to a river of fire. It was a dragon seen close to. A drop of saliva oozed from the dragon's jaws and in the drop was a baby. I took the baby up, or went up myself and the baby reappeared after. I arrived on the ordinary turf, and was in the centre. So I moved to the periphery and the radiant child occupied the centre. It gave its light to the circle of white-bearded, white robed old men, and then disappeared.

'The next day at King Arthur's Hall I saw a picture of the coming of Arthur – a radiant child suspended in a globe was being swept in by the sea into the arms of two men on the left of the picture, the child on the right. The coming of Arthur – the sea-birth in Merlin's cave.

'It seemed a vision of the coming of the Child of Light, but at the same time a transition waking-dream of the passing of the energy of my partner's ovum to the person – Day 20.'

The child is like a magical or spiritual child, a guardian angel. One of the purposes of the psychological and spiritual exercises known as 'magic' is to obtain the knowledge and conversation of the H.G.E. (Holy Guardian Angel). Most of the Orders and Lodges – the most famous and influential of which was the Golden Dawn which flourished from 1886 to 1900 – were devoted to cabalistic magic whose glyph is the Tree of Life; and much of the training was masculinist, hierarchical and competitive, which is why these Orders usually broke up. May we suggest that the secret is of the women, and no secret to them, but something completely accessible and natural? Perhaps we now see a way in which women, not men, acquire that Knowledge and Conversation without artificial training, and can impart its benefits. Perhaps this is the whole purpose of the cycle and of menstruation itself; so that by the time menopause comes we have a secure relation to our spiritual side.

7. Men and Menstruation

Sharing dreams is another way of 'calling each other down' into the unconscious. The dreams told provoke deeper dreams. All contacts with the unconscious have this positive feed-back effect, because we have a basic instinct for wholeness however much society attempts to fragment it. Dreams also are an actuality, and the cycle a mediator between realities.

There are many theories to account for men's fear of menstrual blood. In most aboriginal societies the men acknowledge the women's ability to change their skins like a snake or the moon. This ability is so intolerably dangerous, they say, that if the men don't claim the power of the blood, there will be dislocation of the seasons, weather and crops, as the women cannot be trusted. Despite this, the reports show that in some societies the men's Lodges were learning sensitivity equivalent to the women's through their artificial menstrual rites.[1]

However, the taking-over is more familiar to us in the way in which male-dominated medicine is always telling women the best way to have babies or to menstruate. They seem unable to leave it to women to find things out for themselves, and may even deprive them of the means to do so.

In our society solidarity is simply dismissed. Once the woman takes charge of her cycle and treats it with honour among fellow-women, what are described as distress symptoms begin to modify or fade.

Another theory of the power of the blood is by association with the terrors of birth, the great initial transition and threshold. Blood is the first thing we smell, and we carry that imprint for the rest of our lives. Some psychologists believe that having access to the birth-trauma, through recollections inspired by menstrual blood, is a way of repairing deep layers of the psyche and acquiring new powers.

For the man in the birth encounter, the woman is totally the *other*. A woman comes out of a woman, who came out of a woman, back to the beginning of human time, but a man does not come out of a man, and does not have that primordial community with his own kind. Perhaps that is why he is so anxious to control this *other*.

Nandor Fodor says: 'It is not so much that a woman is unclean in her period but that her bleeding mobilises the pain memories of an archaic dissociation caused by the splitting off of the female from the male.'[2] He is not referring to the birth trauma, though in these words he could be, but rather to the pain of not being a woman. Fodor refers to the idea of a bisexuality lost in the womb by the struggle to become male, but now we know that the reverse happens: the foetus is actually female and the male is produced because of the activity of male hormones. Had these not been present, the child would have been born female.

Ann Belford Ulanov believes that wholeness comes from a female self, in both men and women. Our society is so lacking in femininity, that women in it feel like an 'other' to themselves — and it is the 'other' which completes the personality.[3]

Whatever the theory, it is plain that some men react with great violence against the menstrual cycle. They may become absolutely contrary about it. This is to say, when the woman is in her menstrual state the man can be full of ovulation feelings, and vice versa. He may long for a child during the pre-menstrual time; and he may want the woman to initiate sex at ovulation when that is the time she may want him to be the active partner.

No authority we can find has yet distinguished an autonomous cycle in men. What seems to happen — and it is a view that will not be immediately popular with men — is that men have a physical and mental cycle which reflects the stronger cycle of the woman, and takes an initiatory form parallel to the woman's. As we mentioned in Chapter 1, the famous hero-cycle or 'monomyth' of Joseph Campbell's *The Hero with a Thousand Faces* may originate in the woman's adventurous cyclical sequence of events. However, if the man regards himself as a hero, this may not be mere self-emphasis. It may be because, since he is driven mainly by outside influences and not by an inherent interior cycle, he finds change uncongenial. Indeed, we may find that this resistance to change in the man — to moving from one brain-hemisphere to another, if you like – may be a direct cause of menstrual distress.

The man's initiation cycle may have a shape either *consonant* with the woman's, or one which is *contradictory* and compensatory. That is, his chart can either echo the rhythm of the woman, with transition depression or separation anxiety (and male cravings, often for alcohol, with accompanying hydration too) at the same part of the cycle when she experiences these things; or it may contradict her pattern – when she is clear he is troubled and vice versa. If the man's cycle falls into the same shape as the woman's (including dream-images), her menstrual distress will be considerably reduced. This is a curious fact, difficult to explain. It is as if the man can have a PMS or POS *couvade* (which is the phenomenon by which a man may experience or simulate labour pains when his partner is having a baby). Similarly, it seems, he can get the PMS or POS instead of her. Then *she* sails through this part of the cycle without trouble. Needless to say, this idea is unpopular with many men. But perhaps he, with his ego-resistance to change and transformation, causes at least some of the transition or separation distress. After all, if the woman resists her own changes, she will experience stress and menstrual trouble. So it is quite likely that the mental resistance of her closest partner will also result in trouble. A conscious put-down certainly will; so will an unconscious one. We shall see (pages 96–105) that women tend to move easily between and use both brain-hemispheres, while men don't. This situation could easily be a source of PMS, POS, and of ruined cycles.

If there is a positive relationship between the two, the man, at his good times, can nurse the woman through a cycle 'bump', and vice versa. If the relationship is not so good, then the man is likely to take over the cycle with his complaints, and the woman will feel obliged to tend him and suppress as far as she can her cycle distress (which will then take some other form, probably menstrual irregularity). The man may have contradictory ovulation and family feelings when the woman is in her menstrual state, and inward-going feelings when she is ovulating and needs to enfold *him*. Again, this is likely to lead to menstrual irregularity, like a gyroscope hit off-course with a wobble in its spin.

The source of much of this male disturbance of the cycle will have been his own relationship with the cycle in his infancy. If, as is statistically very likely, his mother suffered from bad transition depression and separation anxiety and a reluctance to accept her period, these moods will have been received by the child. A third of women begin menstruating even while they are breast-feeding. This will be a powerful source of emotion, affecting the child's feeding, for good or ill, depending on the mother's acceptance of the cycle. If she enjoys her period and the transition, then it will be a special time of intimacy; but the usual emotion, especially a generation ago, would have been a mixture of fear of the period and desire for it. Men separate themselves from the period, in the process of separating from the mother, and embrace masculine non-menstruation values. This can be a factor leading to the consciously obstructive reaction, as mentioned above. Yet much creativity will be bound up in this mother-complex, and can be drawn upon by knowing the cycle. The successful negotiation of difficulty in a given cycle is always an initiation into fresh and productive feelings.

Good health generally, assisted, if there is no medical objection, by vitamin and mineral supplementation to offset environmental poisons, is often the first step to improving the individual cycle and its synchrony with a male partner, family or woman friends. Treatment with any supplement or remedy has its subjective and symbolic aspect, besides its physical one. Undoubtedly, taking the right vitamin pill does one good. Also undoubtedly, one is approaching the unknown, as it might be a cave with a lion in it. One has a piece of meat (the vitamin pill) in one hand, and lays it at the cave's mouth. The lion, the unknown, accepts it, and becomes one's friend. Besides the nutritive value of the meat, the giving of it is an act of friendship or even commitment to the unknown, and the unknown responds, kindly. This is where mind and body meet. We recommend that *both* partners take any remedy.

Anthropology shows how men during the course of tribal history have invented rites of shedding magic blood in order to steal magical — that is, political — power from the women and to break up the latter's solidarity. In tribal society no woman is allowed to come near the man's rituals of shedding blood from artificially produced wounds in their bodies. They would by their hilarity break the imitation 'magic' of what comes so naturally to the woman.

In our society the males have instead tabooed and ignored the woman's shedding of blood with the same result: the women lose connection and communication with each other, they lose their solidarity, and menstruation becomes regarded even by women as an anomaly and a sickness.

Restore that solidarity to women and you heal that sickness. At the same time you restore political power. The Australian aborigines were among those societies which believed that if women were allowed to menstruate together, then the world would be overwhelmed by floods and fires and would come to an end.[4] We have suggested that meeting together and discovering menstrual synchrony are powerful solutions to menstrual distress. The world as we know it would indeed come to an end if the women took command of their menstruation and childbirth.

Every person has experienced menstruation as a child. Here lies one of the great puzzles in modern psychology which stresses, on the one hand, that nearly all women suffer from some cyclic disturbances and exert a considerable influence on other people thereby. On the other hand there is a great silence about the contribution this influence makes to the individual child's psychology. This silence is so complete it seems wilful.

The whole movement and atmosphere of the home is cyclical. Children and young people are sensitive to changes in their mother; sometimes she has an unexplained illness; there are days of strain and tension, followed by wonderful relaxation. Blood may be found in the toilet; its smell will be an underlying part of the house's air. The child's psyche, girl or boy, lives according to this rhythm.

A girl eventually develops her own rhythm which is influenced by the mother's. This can happen to an extraordinary extent. One young child lost a milk tooth for six months in succession in synchrony with the mother's period, as though blood had to be shed even though her periods had not yet begun. Losing a tooth is also a frequent pre-menstrual dream image.

A boy, however, never develops a rhythm from his own personal physiology. There are hormone fluctuations in men, for instance in testosterone, but so far nobody seems to have detected a fully-fledged male rhythm, though men are susceptible to a cyclical rhythm, probably learned from mothers and sisters.[5] Children of either sex may begin masturbation during the mother's pre-menstrual phase, to relieve that tension – hence the famous psychoanalytical equation in male psychology between semen and blood. When he comes to live with a woman his response to her periods will be very strongly influenced, consciously or unconsciously, by his experiences of his mother's cycle. In our experience, dreams in men usually show a monthly rhythm, as does body temperature (measured at the same time as the partner's).

Men, as representatives of society's ruling class, will also be influenced by society's willed ignorance of the cycle and its features. Remember, it is the will of society that the majority of women should have no clear picture of their cycles. Not only education but physiology may militate against the man's participation in his partner's changes. His testosterone levels seem to favour left-brain lateralization, and actually direct his mental events away from the right-brain qualities of the menstrual experience. The connection between the two hemispheres is also not so ample as the woman's (for more about this see Chapter 11). Yet his nerve-development and grasp of life is incomplete unless he too makes his adventure and initiation of withdrawal and return and learns to transform, to 'change his skin', as the woman does. It is therefore harder for the man. And as long as he resists participating in her changes, he will be one of the causes of PMS and other cyclical troubles, as his every gesture of body-language will speak against them. His male smell will force the woman to stay in the ovulatory mode longer than she may wish – it has been shown that the presence of men actually shortens the period and promotes ovulation, which means that a male presence, in itself, will delay the transition from ovulation to menstruation. But the pheromone production is responsive to emotion: if the male acquiesces in the changes, a reinforcement to her changes emanates from his body, and this is marked by a slight PMS or POS of his own.

The first practical step is for the man to make a chart of his exhilarations and depressions, using his female partner's cycle-days. Thus both partners make their own menstrual mandalas. He should also record his dreams, again with reference to what is happening in the female cycle. The dream-records should be open to each other, because the sharing of dreams is one of the primary adult bonds, and is healing in itself. He should also take the woman's food supplements and even, with professional advice, her remedies.

This concentration on home-based cyclical time instead of frantic social linear time is difficult in most lives. The question is whether you prefer PMS and POS in the home, with their influence on the relationship and on the children. The discontents of modern marriage are a witness to the ravages that have been visited on the woman's psychology by the age-old wrecking of her cyclical knowledge. It should be through the mother's cycle and home-rhythm that children learn transition from outward to inward mode and back again – outwardly creative to innerly creative, and vice versa – and how there are two sides to every problem, how a solution comes by change of mode, and how to pass on, and let go, in due time, 'moving with change'.

A particular air-borne hormone has been distinguished and isolated, a fatty acid whose effect is to reduce the man's sexuality in the late luteal phase.[6] This is the time of progesterone peak – when a plug against semen is formed in the cervix! The man should not try to manufacture sexual feeling at this time, for this is when non-sexual body-contact is most appreciated in the cycle; a loving touch is sovereign. If it is safely negotiated – it is the time implantation of a fertilized ovum might have occurred – then it is likely to be superseded by the energy of a good pre-menstrual phase, and this energy can be transferred to the partner sexually.

Post-ovulation separation is a time when much menstrual distress is sparked off, continuing thereafter during the pre-menstrual week. It is marked by the peak of the corpus luteum – around Day 21 in a twenty-eight-day cycle – and psychologically, at least, is analogous to the gathering and tensing of the body's resources for a birth. It is in fact not a physical birth, but a birth into a new state. If handled well, one is taken into a clear, energetic pre-menstrual week followed by a good period. If not, a 'domino effect' is liable to fill the subsequent week with pre-menstrual symptoms, started off by a bad handling of the last moments of preparation for possible pregnancy. Around Day 21 may be a threshold of this kind, since by then the cycle *knows* there is going to be no implantation (this is usually achieved around Days 14 to 19) but the corpus luteum is still pouring out progesterone, the pregnancy hormone.

In fact much of the confusion over pre-menstrual syndrome is that it is *two* processes. The first is separation from ovulation, which may cause great stress, as we have described. Then there may be a day or two of quiet, the movement away from ovulation having been achieved. Then comes the second process, pre-menstrual transition, which has its own flavour, quite distinct from the ovulation separation. Without knowledge, these two – separation and transition – may collide, producing a fortnight's distress. If distinguished, it will probably be found that only one of these thresholds causes distress, which therefore limits it to certain days, and shortens it.

It is at this time that the man's couvade can be very effective, if he takes notice of what is happening in himself. He can take on himself as they appear and before they grow, the slight aches and pains in the woman which signal the recession of the corpus luteum, rather like a healer. He will feel them if he acknowledges them, as they act on his hormone-balance, but they will pass through him quite quickly.

He is likely in any case to have slight depression or anxiety, and to accumulate fluid. As above, it is likely to be a lowish time sexually. If he cuddles with plenty of body-contact and, if possible, shared imagery, he may well experience a night of disturbing dreams of such vividness that emerging from them is like a rebirth. The dreams will draw upon childhood times when his mother experienced the ovulation transition, and communicated it to the family. He is likely to lose accumulated water during these hours in sweat and urine (perhaps such nights in childhood led to bed-wetting). But the results should be fresh realizations and balanced energy in both partners during what otherwise might be a dangerous few days. Alternatively, his couvade may be needed in the last few days of the cycle, in the immediate pre-menstrual phase, but it is not likely that it will be needed for both ovulation separation and menstrual transition.

The male partner gives birth to himself, as it were, at this transition, and does this work on behalf of his relationship. Ideally, all the transitions can eventually be experienced in dreaming and waking creativity without physical distress.

Part III

Further Practices

'Alchemy is the science of becoming aware of the whole project in which we are being engaged ... Its name probably means *the art of the black*, and alludes in all likelihood not to the black soil of Egypt but to the black blankness of the unknown brain, the "silent areas" in which the Operator, bent night and day over his fire, eventually kindles a Voice.'

Robert Kelly, 'An Alchemical Journal' in *The Alchemical Tradition in the Late Twentieth Century* (1983)

8. Moon and Weather

The Chinese say that we possess more than one hundred senses, most of them latent. If you saw the BBC television series *Supersense*, you'll be aware that while humans rely on eyesight for much of their information, there are many other ways of perceiving the world.

Guy Murchie in one of his brilliant popular scientific texts[1] distinguishes thirty-two senses, which include sensitivity to radiation other than visible light, such as radio waves, x-rays, gamma rays; temperature sense; the sensing of electro-magnetic fields; awareness of pressure; response to infra- and ultra-sonic frequencies (human beings sometimes get sick in seaside towns due to the reflection of the subsonics of ocean storms from clouds); inner touch, of heartbeat, breathing, blood circulation, which one can also listen to; sense of weight and balance; space or proximity sense; Coriolis sense, awareness of the earth's rotation; appetite, or sensing the state of one's internal organs; humidity sense, which goes with weather sensitivity, as does the sensing of electro-magnetic fields; pain; sense of fear; procreative urges; sense of play; time sense and biological clock, including the menstrual cycle; navigation sense, partly magnetic in humans; and many other complex senses including the spiritual sense of completeness in sacrifice (in dreams menstruation can reveal itself as a kind of 'willing sacrifice') and 'cosmic consciousness'.

For the main part these less-explored senses operate 'underground' and create a living background which rises into consciousness, perhaps as feeling, perhaps in a dream or a change of mood. We are bombarded by these data continually, but we do not for the main part allow them consciousness.

Animals have directly enhanced senses of smell, hearing, taste and touch and even the ability to navigate or seek their food through electrical and magnetic sensory receptors. In this sense, there is something just a bit animal about the menstrual state. Many women find that their senses are enhanced at the premenstrual or menstrual times; these are, however, the 'dark' or non-visual senses of smell, taste, hearing and touch. Women are better endowed with these non-visual senses than men are; women are most acutely visual at their ovulation.

PMS and POS sufferers often feel that smells become too harsh or disturbing, sensitivity to noise increases and there is also a sharp reaction to 'atmospheres', bad or good 'vibes'. The pre-menstrual person feels that she has lost a skin, and is accordingly too sensitive. One cannot say that this is the cause of POS or PMS but it is certainly an important factor. However, once the menstrual state is reached, especially if there is some creative outlet, this increased vividness of experience finds its harmonies. While such resolutions can happen in the pre-menstrual state, too often it is jangling instead. The inner senses, the sense of one's body, one's organs and bones, are stimulated too, so that touch and hearing, taste and smell may make their appearance in the dreams of a dreamer who is usually mostly visual. If one smells something in a dream one can be sure that a resolution of some conflict has begun or is completed. There may be entirely non-visual dreams, which can be frightening until one gets used to them. On entering the menstrual state there may be 'lucid' dreams in which one is aware one is dreaming, but is possessed of one's usual senses; this kind of dream may bring revelation, like a visionary or religious experience. With the inner senses operating, autoscopy is likely to occur: that is, the seeing-within of some organ or function of the body. A relaxed breath may be visualized as a swooping flight of birds, indigestion as a sharp sword piercing the belly, and pre-menstrual fluid accumulation in the legs as wearing a heavy pair of wellington boots and wading through water. It is a frequent dream that the period has come, and to wake and find it has.

That is internal environment. But sensitivity at PMS, POS, or any other time, to external environment is one of the great neglected areas of common human experience, like the menstrual cycle itself. The upset and stress we experience with weather-changes are some of the tattered remnants of our erstwhile continuum with nature, which was in other ages mediated through women's sensitivity and weather wisdom.

A menstrual or pre-menstrual person should ally herself with these intuitions. The environment is packed with stimuli which, in our primarily visual way, we ignore to our cost. The most ancient of these intuitions is that the women's cycle has a relationship to the phases of the moon. Many women will admit to talking to the moon, perhaps from before their first period, asking, 'When will it come? When?' The moon certainly in her tides influences all living organisms in the wild, and reaches women through that sensitive rhythmic process we call the menstrual cycle, even in the cities. Women moving house to the seaside often find that their periods have naturally entrained with the lunar month; using a menstrual mandala marked with the moon phases may aid the act of attention which can so synchronize the cycle. Traditionally women were supposed to menstruate on the new moon or in the dark of the moon (that is to say, when the moon rises with the sun, hidden in its light) and to ovulate on the full moon, the phase during which fertility ceremonies were usually performed. Some women find that their cycles move round so that menstruation occurs either at full or new moon, and that the two cycles have different feelings: perhaps more motherly with the full-moon ovulation, and more imaginatively creative (this goes with the enhancement of the 'dark' senses, called by Freud 'primary process') with the full-moon menstruation. Many 'irregularities' of the cycle may actually be meaningful adjustments, but until every woman keeps her menstrual mandala we cannot expect the subject to be fully known. It is pioneer work which each woman who starts a chart as both map-guide and symbolic instrument takes part in for the benefit of all.

The oldest calendar markings known are moon-markings and they were menstrual calendars also. The oldest symbol known is the wheel cross, and this is a pattern of the moon's phases, which for many people provides the simplest and most accurate menstrual mandala.

Though the moon moves contrary to the sun against the background of stars, we have preferred in our charts to mark the progress of the phases as on the face of a clock, as time moves in that direction, from past to present. Some ancient monuments show the whole moon cycle in relation to the position of the earth by the same 'wheel cross'.

A *symbol* collects dreams; this is why the menstrual mandala encourages dream recall, and, above all, reveals the basic narrative behind the dream-sequences of the child-bearing years. There is an old saying in Latin: *In habentibus symbolum facilior est transitus* meaning 'For those who have a symbol it is easier to change'. These ancient symbolic or right-brain patterns are psychologically effective in present times. Many people with an approximately lunar cycle of around twenty-eight days (on which we have based our diagrams) can relate that cycle to the moon's, and pattern it in a very similar way to the wheel cross.

Many people's cycles seem to fall into this four-fold pattern quite naturally, with or without lunar synchrony. If the cycle is longer or shorter, that is usually said to be due to variation in the first fortnight. Thus people can often succeed in adjusting the cycle by sleeping with an indirect light on at about the thirteenth, fourteenth and fifteenth days (a lamp shielded so it shines gently, like moonlight, from a white ceiling is appropriate); if one does this, then the period is quite likely to arrive a fortnight later. Many people discover that distinguishing the four directions like this (like 'boxing the compass' or 'squaring the circle') does give them their basic pattern. Dreams often follow this sequence.

Once you start dreaming seriously, scary things may happen, especially in pre-menstrual times. Remember, if you dream an image, you possess it now, it doesn't possess you. So take courage. A dream-recorded ovulation seldom goes by without one's seeing *round* objects: a round table, an egg, a football (rugby football with its oval projectile is a frequent dream-image at ovulation), a glittering diamond earring hanging from *one* ear.

Then again, dreams at menstruation or shortly before often show images of the womb itself. Sometimes these are feral: the womb's energies can appear as animals, a fox or a wolf, and the round, muzzled heads with the pricked-up ears resemble the structure of the womb. A horned animal, like a cow or a goat, shows the Fallopian tubes sweeping up, and one may even meet and converse, as it were, with one's own womb in the image of a horned god. This of course was the mediaeval image of the Devil consorting with witches, and such dreams may be the truth behind the persecutions and martyrdom of women in the Middle Ages.

The influence of the weather on the menstrual cycle is profound or – to put it another way – the amount of information about the environment one can pick up by being attentive to one's menstrual cycle is almost limitless. We humans do have those extra senses.

Until they are trained, a person may notice only how terrible they feel if, for example, the pre-menstrual time coincides with the moving in of cold fronts. About 30 per cent of the population suffer from extreme weather-sensitivity to the point of illness. Women are more susceptible to weather changes than men, simply because their constitution is linked to those same balances of neuro-transmitters and hormones as are responsible for the self-expression of the menstrual cycle.

The greatest sensitivity to weather will occur at those times when other distress is felt, and contributes to that distress. Weather sensitivity is interestingly similar to PMS symptoms. People become witchy and moody, have attacks of nerves, become uncoordinated for no apparent reason. Sulman's aphorism on sensitivity to weather electricity could apply as well to PMS and POS: 'We do great injustice to the electro-sensitive patients, who rightly complain of their serotonin sufferings, when we treat them as psychiatric patients. They have a sixth sense that makes them suffer and therefore deserve our help.' That 'sixth sense' is part of menstrual sensitivity. And, yes, human beings are sensitive to electricity, especially weather electricity.[2]

It can be as difficult being moved by the weather from a high-pressure system to a low-pressure system as being moved, by the cycle, from ovulation to menstruation. The two extremes are contrary opposites. Some people operate better in high barometric pressure, others in low. The high-pressure system is an immense swirl or maelstrom of spinning clouds and waves or steps of barometric pressure running with immense power *clockwise*. High-pressure systems suit the majority of human beings, that is, if they don't go on too long. If they do, the electrical fields grow too tense for us, especially when there is a likelihood of thunder-storms. Low-pressure systems are perhaps less well tolerated, to an extent that may depend on your phase of the cycle. Many people experience a depression during the arrival of a cold front and a weather depression – a vast swirling *anti-clockwise* dynamo generating immense currents. Transition from a very high-pressure system to a low could bring the period on. The walls of the womb are very delicate at this time and a change in barometric pressure from, say, 1030 millibars to 984, would be enough to stimulate the bleeding. This can feel like a wonderful communion with nature, outside with inside. Weather, it should be noted, is also linked to lunar-phases. The two opposing high-pressure, low-pressure wheels of air as they touch each other interact. The word is an understatement: they fight and wrestle like coiling serpents, or like chain-saws fighting. Tremendous electrical forces are released. Human beings, with their congenital power of being able to tamp back most things they don't want to know into unconsciousness, manage to ignore these forces. That the body does not in fact ignore them can be shown in the lab by urine and blood analysis: the constituents fluctuate as wildly as the weather itself.

The people who can't ignore these fluctuations, the weather-sensitive, can feel cold fronts – that is, the movement of a low-pressure system into a high-pressure one – a couple of hundred miles away. Those who have wounds or scars, particularly amputees, can also feel and predict the weather in advance. Women, who have a 'Wise Wound' are usually weather-sensitive, but because they are more used to 'inner weather' than men are, they are able to carry on. But people with difficult menstrual thresholds will have difficult weather thresholds and the two may often coincide, causing exquisite sensitivity to weather. On the physical, measurable, level there will be fluctuating neuro-transmitters and the swelling of hydration, which turns a person into a kind of pressure-sensitive barometer. The pressure reaction causes fingers to swell and rings to tighten before storms; they tighten too, of course, during the pre-menstrual phase. People who are menstruating may respond to cold fronts and storms with cramps; the great inner wound and scar-tissue of the lining of the womb in menstruation can be as sensitive as an amputation. The person with pre-ovulation tension is also likely to be sensitive, but to a lesser degree. As a cold front tunnels into the warm face of air it is penetrating the whirling masses of air, mixing moist and cold, generating tremendous electrical tension, as if the air were hands rubbing the fur of an immense black thunder-cloud sky-cat.

Human beings respond to these changes at all times with minute but measurable alterations of their inner chemical and electrical environment. The electrical configuration of the skies is reflected by movements of electricity within the soil, rocks and the earth's surface generally, and this will include electrical events within the cage of water-pipes and wiring that are our houses; people who are sensitive will respond, and how sensitive you are depends upon many things including your present station in the menstrual cycle.

The weather is a tremendous input of environmental information that most of us either put into the unconscious mind (where it may form symbols experienced in dreams) or perceive as illness, as we perceive the unsymbolized changes of the menstrual cycle's inner weather as sickness. It is the *change* from one weather to another which is agonizing – another parallel with the cycle.

Theoretically this sensitivity could be that 'sixth sense' which would give a person 'magical' knowledge of the world. If one records dreams, it will be found that there are weather-dreams which reflect actual weather conditions. You can add weather to your menstrual mandala parameters, and keep a watch for, say, cold fronts with the aid of the weather-charts from newspapers. In this way you can watch how your menstrual cycle reacts, and thus bring this important environmental sense to consciousness.

People who do yoga and the like can tell by the flexibility of their joints and the depth of their yoga-breathing what the weather is likely to be that evening or tomorrow. Yoga and Do-In (oriental self-massage) assist in adjusting to the weather. Nutritional supplements can also help, exactly as they help the cycle which may shorten or lengthen in response to weather-stress, as it may to the seasons. The mandala kept over the months will reveal this. Homoeopathy knows a great deal about weather sensitivity, which will be part of your homoeopathic clinical picture.

Once, 'wise women' gave their community advice on the time to plant crops or to harvest. This inner knowledge must have derived partly from weather-sensitivity, sensitivity that the modern person can experience by studying the menstrual cycle. A knowledge of the symbolizations that weather elicits in dreams and visions would have been part of that knowledge. The men would then be spurred to outward observation, lacking the cycle's sensitivity.

Anybody can try an experiment on these lines with no more than simple aspirin. Aspirin was originally derived from the willow, which of course grows in damp places very responsive to weather. It was a remedy from earliest times for weather aches and pains. If you feel that bad weather is coming, and you ache, take some aspirin and have a short rest and a sleep. Not only will the aches be eased, but you will probably get a dream to go with it that will cheer you up.

One of the most easily measurable and accountable of environmental electrical influences is the presence or absence of negative ions. Remember how oppressive the build-up of a thunder-cloud feels, especially if one is directly underneath it. This is due to the tremendous escalating electrical forces in the cloud, which is negatively charged overall, inducing a positive charge on you and the ground beneath. This positive charge feels unnatural and unpleasant because the earth is usually negatively charged. When the rain falls there is a wonderful refreshment of the air and one tingles with life and sensuous intelligence. This is because the negative charge has now been carried downwards.

Negative ion generators are now plentifully on the market in inexpensive versions, and they can transform your home environment. They help pass both weather and menstrual thresholds, especially if there is an interaction between your cycle and the weather. They are simply good to have on, as they make the air feel crisp and lively. If at pre-menstrual time you and your family suffer from the sniffles, an ionizer will usually improve the situation quite remarkably. It tends to produce a stable field in a room while the weather is fluctuating wildly outside; so does a coal fire or a lighted candle. Negative ionization also appeals to the 'dark' senses as it increases the sensitivity of the skin. The manufacturer's instructions should be carefully followed, and one should be chosen which guarantees the right load per emitter and hence no ozone.

Another strategy for improving inner weather really belongs to seasonal changes, which are also mixed up with cycle response. Doctors are beginning to recognize a condition known as Seasonal Affective Disorder (SAD). Anyone who suffers from this grows exceedingly depressed due to the reduction of light in the winter. The cure is a bank of fluorescent tubes simulating daylight, in whose light the patient sits. Ordinary electric lights do not provide a full sunlight spectrum. This apparatus is expensive, but is needed for full-scale winter depression.

Fortunately there are much cheaper daylight simulation bulbs which are more expensive than ordinary bulbs, but not prohibitively so, and which will supply some of the lacking light-nourishment, and raise the spirits in winter months if used as illumination in key positions.

The violent discontinuities which the weather can produce are rather like the amnesias in the cycle itself. In its individual rhythm the menstrual cycle is an entry to the massive rhythms of nature neglected in our society as a direct influence on our lives.

Damp places in particular communicate weather changes to humans. This is true of the home. If you live in a damp place with varying and difficult weather, then it is well worth investing in a dehumidifying machine which will take the excess moisture from the air and keep it at an optimum level. This is good for the health of the house as well as of the people within it. One can say goodbye to water-streaming window panes and damp smells from books or carpets. An optimum humidity will also enliven the air and the sense of touch, thus aiding the 'passing of thresholds'. Like the ionizer, it helps to maintain a stable atmosphere in the house. In such a stable atmosphere one tends to become more sensitive to changes of feeling in the people one is sharing the house with. Most electrical shops now sell efficient and quiet dehumidifiers.

There is a neat little device that adjusts body sensitivity to weather currents, and can produce powerful stimulation or deep tranquillity. This is the Eeman circuit. Measurable polarities exist in various parts of the body, and change according to the menstrual cycle (there is one device for measuring fertility through skin resistance), and this simple circuit may be a way of adjusting or equalizing them, and allowing them to flow. Note any images in the reverie, as in post-coital relaxation, and relate to the cycle.

The Eeman circuit (so called after L. E. Eeman who had a distinguished Harley Street practice in the 1940s and described his results in a remarkable book, *Co-Operative Healing*) is easy to make.[3] You need two squares of fine copper gauze to which are attached long wires, preferably with copper terminals. Wearing ordinary clothes, you simply lie down with one screen behind your head and the other under the base of your spine, holding the head terminal in the left hand and the other in your right hand. That is the relaxation circuit, and it is liable to send you to sleep.

Reversing the terminals sets up another circuit which reinforces the tension of the polarities between head and pelvis, and can stimulate you like a cup of coffee, though, like coffee, it can make you irritable.

You should cross your left ankle over your right. Usually right-handedness doesn't affect the basic circuit, but there is a small proportion of people in which the polarity is reversed, and this can be adjusted by experiment. Instead of copper gauze, try pads of silk with silk strips instead of the linking wires.[4]

Link up two partners, and you will get the impression of sharing pre-menstrual energy, if it is that time of the month, and of post-coital relaxation without actually having sex. Children also respond well.

When the circuit works, you can feel a soothing pulse through the whole body; yes, this could be imagination, but if so, allow the imagination to co-operate. The circuit can relieve low back pain, whether or not this occurs during a pre-menstrual time. If the circuit works for you, you can experiment with all kinds of ways of linking it up, as Eeman did, with considerable success. There are indications that a woman with pre-menstrual energy could share it with several people with healing results; rather like Mesmer's salons where people apparently took 'animal magnetism' like taking the waters at a spa!

Unless you feel an affinity with polarity healing, and have had a good experience of it, these ideas may seem too speculative. You should approach these practices with 'a willing suspension of disbelief'. Rough scepticism will simply untune your attention. We are partners with these natural forces, not their bosses.

9. A Note on Rhythm

We are creatures of rhythm: of the rhythm of the seasons, of day and night, of the many minute rhythms of the cell, the sea, the air, and of the environment at large. The menstrual rhythm is the pulse that connects us to nature's rhythms: it is a kind of complex aggregate of all the rhythms that affect us, focusing in a simple four-fold form. In a sense it is like a gyroscope that spins true however much the ship is rocking, but a simple abrupt shove will break up the spin and, tracing many wobbly patterns, the wheel will fall on its side. This is what happens to the menstrual cycle that is abused by its taboo; it also happens to bicyclists who don't believe in themselves – they wobble and fall off.

Everything has its own particular and individual resonance and harmony. It is easy to visualize this by considering water and land under the tides of the moon.

> The individual nature of a stretch of water is expressed in the waves which vibrate in it and vibrate in various harmonies and rhythms. To the peculiar nature of a stretch of water belongs also an individual movement which fluctuates with a slower, more extended rhythm, while bearing on its surface the more delicate play of waves caused by the wind. Every water basin, whether ocean, lake or pond, has its own natural period of vibration. This varies according to the shape, size and depth of the basin. The whole morphological character of a lake finds expression in this natural period of vibration; it is like a 'note' to which the lake is 'tuned'. This 'note' has 'overtones' in its vibration, like a flute or the string of a musical instrument ... The natural period of vibration of a stretch of water is in more or less marked resonance with the path of the moon and its tide producing forces. The resonance is

strongest when the natural period of vibration corresponds to the orbital rhythm of the moon ... As the moon wanders over the different waters of the earth, they respond to a greater or lesser degree with their 'note' according to how closely their natural period of vibration is tuned to the rhythm of the moon. All together they are like a great musical instrument, spread out over the earth, on which the moon plays an inaudible melody, which wanders with it round the earth.[1]

Everybody has observed the workings of this visible music. In it we can see the rhythmic play of the environment, and how each being responds in its own resonance to the greater rhythms. This is an interaction that runs through the whole universe, from the greatest to the smallest:

If in a long view of the ocean, say, one could regard the tides as nothing but extremely long, low ocean waves of a super order and very slow period, so might the end waves of radiation be conceptually extended into other orders of space and time: down into the deep infra-bass frequencies of slow-flashing variable stars and whole gyrating galaxies, and – why not? – up into the still less understood ultra-altissimo frequencies that quite possibly vibrate somewhere far inside the inmost hearts of atomic nuclei.[2]

The menstrual cycle, properly considered, can be seen as the human dimension of this hierarchy of tides. In technical terms, it is an oscillator: it vibrates. If oscillators are allowed to vibrate together they entrain, and rhythmic interactions move towards an overall harmony. An oscillator is any object that moves in a regular, periodic manner, anything which vibrates. Everybody knows, again, that piano strings vibrate to their resonant frequency; or, if two violins are tuned, and one put on the table and a note played on the other, we see that the same string that we are playing on one violin is also humming on the other. There is sympathetic resonance between them.

In the same way, if you have several pendulum clocks hanging on a wall, and you start them out of phase with each other, in a day or two they are all beating in phase, locked into rhythm. Something similar happens among women living together, since their menstrual cycles begin to synchronize, like a system of oscillators tuning to each other. This may happen by the rhythmic secretion of airborne hormones ('pheromones'), or the subtle electrical changes that occur in a woman's body, or more likely by the emergence and reinforcement of one big beat from very many subtle factors, including, it is possible, lunar rhythms and cross-sensitivity to ordinary body-language. It is as though by rhythm entrainment the women have become one body or one spirit.

It is curious that science has abstracted this type of system and made it the basis of all television and radio communication, where it is known as the tuned circuit. It is drawn directly from nature, though no doubt unconsciously. The broadcasting oscillator sends out a carrier wave which is simply a featureless rhythm. The receiving oscillator is tuned to this carrier wave. On to the carrier wave is then written, as it were, the broadcast – as a big wave of the ocean may carry surf and surfers and small currents engraved on its sides. Picked up by the receiver oscillator these produce variations in the basic rhythm; the wave carries features which by themselves could not have reached shore, like the surfers. This is how an oscillator – or any rhythmic system – picks up information from the environment. Later in the circuit-system the carrier is cancelled, leaving behind only the information. As the human body is not just electromagnetic, like the radio set (though it is that too), but also electrical, magnetic and chemical, as well as being audibly vibrant and in motion all the time, with every cell and organ being mutually tuning oscillators, surrounded by the whole of nature which is similarly active, there is a lot of information to be picked up. Our ordinary senses are oscillators tuned, for example, to the vibrations of visible light; but we have many more than the visual sense. All our rhythms are sources of knowledge, capable of carrying information at every level. The day and the night go by in their pulses, and engraved on that rhythm are all the events of our day. We resonate to those events, or not, as the case may be. The menstrual rhythm is similarly engraved with many events which it is possible for us to discern. Because the menstrual rhythm, like the heart-beat and the breath, is a rhythm of the whole body, it is one of those core-rhythms which can pick up total information.

If a bodily-environmental rhythm is altered by compulsion, then distress ensues. Most people know something of that interference with the day–night or circadian rhythm we call 'jet-lag'. Its symptoms are very like those of PMS, and may indeed result from a similar imbalance of various hormones and secretions (including the important neuro-transmitter 5HT or serotonin) which may give rise to discomfort as apparently wide apart as PMS, weather sensitivity, or feelings experienced when giving up cigarettes. These chemicals are involved in very complicated metabolic pathways, many of which rely on the supply of a particular nutrient. Under stress, or interference with the body's rhythms, which is also a kind of stress, such nutrients are more rapidly depleted than normal, and lead to neuro-hormone imbalance. Such stress can come also from anxiety due to purely mental sources.

We are dealing with a kind of circulation here between mind and body, psyche and soma. What we call body and what we call mind are, as it were, part of a circulatory system: mind nourishes body, body nourishes mind. It is not possible to speak of the beginning or end of a circulatory system. The unity and interdependence of bodily and mental events were and are pulled apart by the ghost-in-the-machine Cartesian philosophy. But the body is no machine. It is ourselves. Descartes said, 'I think, therefore I am', and made the intellect paramount. But the intellect is the world quartered: every woman can say also 'I feel, therefore I am', 'I sense, therefore I am', 'I intuit therefore I am', and thus by tracing out this four-fold pattern restores an original felt unity with herself and the world.

Working with the menstrual cycle is one way of restoring what has been pulled apart. The dream experience of the cycle is the cycle experience of the dream. The psyche–soma split is healed by the bodily events which reflect the dream, and the dream events which reflect the bodily ones.

10. Discarding the Negative

Negative expectation can be almost the whole problem. If you are asked to fill out a menstrual chart, it will usually be some form of clinical chart, very rectilinear, on which you record entirely negative symptoms. On the face of it this is OK, as you want to rid yourself of those symptoms and they are the events that are to be looked at. As a whole picture of the cycle it can be a failure. The many positive features of the cycle will be missed and, worse, this negative expectation will actually bring about a feed-back effect; noticing only the unpleasant incidents will increase not only their significance but also their occurrence. At times of 'arousal' expectation can create the phenomenon. An injection of plain distilled water can be given in gloomy circumstances and the 'injection' will 'depress', but the same water can be injected with the promise that it is a stimulant, and then the subject is inclined to get high. This is one of the most significant features of the menstrual cycle, that it is rather like a genie's lamp; ask of it and it will give what is needed. Genius lamp.

The pre-menstrual state is not necessarily in itself a bad time, even in people with strong reactions to it. It can be a state of heightened ability, as, indeed, can any other part of the cycle. Dr Michelle Harrison, in a recent book, says:

> [PMS] in some ways resembles a heightened state of consciousness, an experience of being in a different world, of looking at life through a magnifying glass. It is often a world with its own internal consistency. Some women describe an enhancement of creativity and perceptiveness, a richness of sensation and imagery lacking at other times.[1]

It is clear that Dr Harrison is speaking of a PMS that has found its mental dimension, and does not merely exist and suffer in the physical world. She quotes a woman sculptor: 'There is a quality to my work and to my vision which just isn't there the rest of the month. I look forward to being pre-menstrual for its effect on my creativity, although some of the other symptoms create strains with my family.'

Dr Harrison's book contains useful advice about charts, though she does not distinguish different components of distress that begins at ovulation, all of which she describes as 'pre-menstrual'. She does, however, emphasize the positive and creative events that can occur during these times.

The sculptor is a woman who has found the creative dimension of the menstrual energies, and insists on their being taken on their own terms. If one finds this periodical access of energy, it is wise to arrange for some work to be ready to be taken up at that precise time of the month. This post-ovulation 'high' time may signal a successful ovulation-separation. If this happens in the last few pre-menstrual days, after recession of the corpus luteum, this energy will be the flipside of pre-menstrual distress. Both these favourable times could be there for all women, except that there is such a negative expectation of the period and all that precedes it.

Dr Harrison also quotes the words of a woman subject to that depression, which she sees as the cost of a certain achievement: 'When I am premenstrual I can write with such clarity and depth that after I get my period I don't recognise that those were my thoughts or that I could have written anything so profound.' Clearly this woman has, through recognizing and honouring a feared time of the cycle, opened up communications with her hitherto unknown self. A very handy way of doing this we will describe later, under the heading of 'sealed writing' (see pages 144–5).

Dr Harrison, who is a noted physician dealing exclusively with PMS in her practice, points in the direction of what we have called right-brain facility manifested in the pre-menstrual time. She quotes other women: 'I feel receptive premenstrually, and more sensitive, I take everything in but I can't discriminate well. Then later I have to try to figure it all out.' This is certainly one of the states of creativity, when all you wanted pours out. On no account should one stop it while it is coming. One can trim and discriminate later, using one's left brain at a different stage of the cycle. 'Invent a jungle, and *then* explore it.' If you haven't allowed the jungle to grow first then there will be nothing to explore. But women are discouraged from using this transition time when it turns out to be productive, and then, feeling the pressure of unexpressed creativity, protest in body language of illness.

In other women the period itself seems to have a balancing function. 'I get scared I'll get lost in my work. I'm in a frenzy with it and then I get my period and I'm different again.' 'For me sexual energy and creative energy seem to come at the same time in my cycle. For a while I'm driven crazy by both but I get a lot done and then I menstruate and I feel normal again.' This confirms again that the transition time can be an important threshold that can be passed consciously.

Dr Harrison comments:

> Women may have a lessening of boundaries, of control and rules during the pre-menstrual time. *They seem to be directed more by what is occurring internally than externally* ... Along with the lessening of constraint, there is also a heightened sensitivity to sound, sight and smell. Colours may take on a different hue.

She says: 'The ability to put expression into form is not improved during the premenstrual time.' In other words, a writer may write well pre-menstrually but edit well after her period. An artist said: 'I do sketches when I am premenstrual. That's when I get my ideas, but I never start the full drawing then. I can't get the lines the way I want them. I see them, but I can't do it right on paper.' Then it is right brain before the period in her case, and left brain co-operates afterwards. Boundaries melt and flow at the pre-menstrual transition time and some react to this as a threat to the ego and the accepted world, with all gradations of sickness from the madness of disbelief in oneself down to the involuntary self-rejection of an allergy or an auto-immune reaction.

Dr Harrison names a condition she calls Pre-menstrual Magnification (PMM). This is when an illness becomes worse pre-menstrually. She says: 'PMM, like PMS, can be mild and barely noticeable or severe and incapacitating. The magnification can also be one of joy, excitement or creativity.' Such magnification can happen at any time of arousal, pre-ovulatory, for example. But the capacity of the creative or transition side of PMS to take one into unexplored territories of oneself, can also offer opportunities for curing an illness not immediately related to the cycle, but magnified by a sensitive or vulnerable part of it. Then an illness which recurs may become subject to the dream process, and find its cure through dream-events and images. This PMM contributes to the 'domino effect', when distress originating in one part of the cycle overflows to other parts.

It is good to leave caches over the cycle for the appropriate time next month. To close up one's pre-menstrual books until the next pre-menstrual time revives them. Many of us forget what one was at a certain time in the cycle. This amnesia is a kind of threshold-shock. Keep work done in a certain time to be picked up when that time comes again.

If PMS accumulates water, and there is a creative effort or profound sex at this time, the water may be shed, and creative energy takes its place. Then the menstrual bleeding arrives as a kind of crown or restful culmination of this work. During the post-ovulation time there are many distractions to negotiate. 'Sniffles' is one. This may not be a cold brought on by the stress found in the cycle (which is energy under another aspect, if it finds its task), but rather a swelling of the mucous membranes as a part of the hydration. Surprisingly, this is one of the effects that can be communicated to others, probably by pheromone action. As one of Dr Harrison's mothers remarks: 'When I have PMS we all have PMS.' Lesbian partners, she points out, may synchronize their cycles, and then the PMS energy can be destructive as 'the tensions, strains and potential for explosions are even greater'; but there may also be like perils of synchrony in the family with daughters growing up.

The tremendous depression and persecutory anxiety experienced before beginning any creative work are familiar to any practising artist. Naturally the lay person suffers in this way, but what we call 'art' is also a way of navigation, available to everybody. Every person must fulfil their creative potential. The artist should be a kind of leader in exploring these unknown areas that communicate with us in PMS and other disturbances. Many women artists are now doing this, instead of building on male ideas of art. Their works will undoubtedly help women navigate the cycle. It is good for women to look at the works of women artists, and use their works to pass thresholds. It is like taking an effigy of the birth-goddess to stand by your bed to help labour.

The sequence in creativity of moods and events is very close to the idea of passing the menstrual thresholds – it may even be the same process. Since art has for so long been a masculine subject, the menstrual analogies with the creative process have been concealed. There is first anxiety and depression, attacks of obligation, splintering and fragmentation, exactly the anxiety-depression picture of the major forms of PMS. Then there is a breakthrough into a state in which ideas come freely, even an 'oceanic' state in which one feels kinship with all things. Clearly, this is like accounts of a good premenstrual transition. Then there is the editing stage, where one no longer feels the exultation directly, but rather establishes it firmly in those parts of the cycle that need it. Then, as the cycle comes round, one may dip again into one's creative well. It is as difficult and rewarding to move from right brain to left brain and vice versa as it is to move from menstruation to ovulation and ovulation to menstruation. In due course the two opposites can fuse and create a new spirit in the menstruatrix – perhaps anticipating the dynamic androgyny of the menopausa. This pattern of descent and return, which we have called the pattern of initiation, may be the basic creative process, felt, suffered and appreciated in its entirety by women in their cycle, which is then reflected in the men, and teaches them creativity. Unfortunately few have acknowledged the debt.

11. Brain Opposites

The idea of 'left brain' and 'right brain' is a useful model for understanding the contrast between two modes of thinking and between the ovulation and the menstruation experiences. Here is a list of qualities that have been almost universally attributed to left and right sides, to left-handedness and right-handedness. Remember, the left brain communicates with the right side of the body, and the right brain the left; there is a cross-over (but not in the ears).

In this list, everything which is despised, mysterious, polluted, feminine, is related to the left-hand side, the sinister side (right brain); and everything which is visible, open, tribally approved, is related to the dexter, right-hand side (left brain). This is a cross-cultural difference which is found in some form or other in every human culture. What is also found in every human culture is an association of the left hand, the polluted, the sinister, the witch-like, with the menstrual experience.

Left Hand – Right Brain	*Right Hand – Left Brain*
Introvert	Extrovert
Wrong	Right
Secret	Public
Sinister	Dexter
Meditation	Action
Female	Male
Evil	Good
Satan	God
Dream world	Actual world
Unconscious	Conscious
Participation	Competition
Poison	Medicine
Accepts	Rejects

BRAIN OPPOSITES

Sickness	Health
Satisfaction	Needs
Hell	Heaven
Spiral	Linear
Belief	Criticism
Moon	Sun
Night	Day
Symbolic	Literal
Implicit	Explicit
Impure	Pure
Primary process	Secondary process
Witch	Priest
Black magician	White magician
Left-hand path	Right-hand path
Implicate order	Explicate order
Sensuous	Intellectual
Polluted	Pure
Eternal return	Straight-line time
Eternity	History
Intuitive	Intellectual
Being	Doing
Mysterious	Open
Dark (non-visual)	Light (visualization)
Despised	Celebrated
Wife	Husband
Self	Tribe
Flow	Containment
Magic	Science
Sublime	Beautiful
Improvization	Calculation

Associated with the right hand (left brain) are family and tribal values, public fame and influence, everything fair, square and above board, these being the values of ovulation. Cross-culturally, too, the woman being the bearer of the apparent contradictions inherent in the cycle is regarded as a dangerous natural force, to be carefully controlled and contained within the rules of 'normality'.

Right-handedness and left-handedness certainly go with the specialization of the brain-hemispheres. What is tabooed is the magic, intuitional, creative and sinister right hemisphere. This taboo and suspicion of the right brain by the left brain resembles the suspicion ovulation has of menstruation; society attempts to squash the bearer of these gifts, the menstruous woman, by denying that menstruation is anything but a sickness.

Just as left-brain science views magic as dangerous self-delusion, so does right-brain creativity view science as that destructive explanatory study which puts the light of the rainbow out. Likewise, ovulation's view of menstruation is that it is the death and cannibalization of children, while menstruation's of ovulation is that it is a stifling family straitjacket and the death of individuality. These conflicts are echoed in developed dream imagery, and provide a guide to the dream process in its progress towards a unification where these conflicts are overcome and the cycle knows itself as a whole. Then the woman no longer suffers those attacks on her nature by her other side (of menstruation by ovulation and vice versa) which results in those conditions known as cycle distress. PMS is an attack on menstruation by ovulation, and pre-ovulatory distress is an attack on ovulation by menstruation; just as the right-brain artist may misunderstand and disparage the left-brain scientist, and vice versa.

Of course the ideal is a balanced attitude. Here is a rumination by a scientist — therefore a predominantly left-brain man — rather grudgingly accepting the gifts of his right-hand brain and understanding how they are complementary to each other. This account could also be what we might imagine a science-educated woman, the mother of children now growing up, would say as she begins to realize the gifts which exist in the menstrual state withheld from her by taboo, yet natural to women. Now ovulation is less important, the other half of the cycle opens to her, and her PMS — fear of the menstrual state — recedes.

> Since childhood, I have been enchanted by the fact and the symbolism of the right hand and the left — the one the doer, the other the dreamer. The right is order and lawfulness, *le droit*. Its beauties are those of geometry and taut implication. Reaching for knowledge with the right hand is science. Yet to say only that much of science is to overlook one of its excitements, for the great hypotheses of science are gifts carried in the left.

Of the left hand we say that it is awkward and, while it has been proposed that art students can seduce their proper hand to more expressiveness by drawing first with the left, we nonetheless suspect this function ... And should we say that reaching for knowledge with the left hand is art? ... It is an approach whose medium of exchange seems to be the metaphor paid out by the left hand. It is a way that grows happy hunches and lucky guesses, that is stirred into connective activity by the poet and necromancer looking sidewise rather than directly. Their hunches and intuitions generate a grammar of their own – searching out connections, suggesting similarities, weaving ideas loosely in a trial web.[1]

However, it now seems that the upshot of left-brain, right-brain research, is that strict lateralization is a kind of mutation that happened to men. It caused them to favour the right-handed, left-brained values of control, manipulation and linear logic, and consequently to favour the ovulation side of the cycle which loves to control nature, providing, as it were, the admass for manipulation. The motherhood role has therefore been over-cultivated. The other side of things, the sinister, right-brain capabilities, seem tucked away in the unconscious mind, in the much diminished, much tabooed functions of menstruation and right-brain artistic acts. Creativity is as great a taboo as menstruation is.

Roberto Assagioli uses the metaphor of a marriage to discuss the relationship between analytical mind and intuition.

First, there is a good number of those who do not even contemplate such a marriage. They are content to either use only the intuitive or only the intellect ... in some cases one of the partners is too imperative and devaluates and keeps in subjection the other – and it can be either one that makes this mistake, with all the drawbacks of repression, of overt or covert rebellion. In other cases there is an oscillation, a fight between the two in which temporarily the one or the other predominates.[2]

This is very much like a real marriage, with the male partner exasperated and the female in the grip of PMS or POS. But, please note, the metaphor itself is masculine. The masculine mind has already been lateralized, or by its attitude actually creates the division between intuition and intellect. This intellect creates itself out of separation.

The consensus of opinion is that the hemispheres of women and men are differently organized, just as their bodily rhythms are. The female cycle has been violently organized *from outside*, as has the brain function, and this is a cause of *menstrual* disjunction and distress, just as organization from outside has been a cause of the repression of feminine culture and *mental* disjunction and distress. Body and mind are complete and not to be separated. The menstrual persecution and the mental persecution are mirror-images. Here we have a model of how male lateralization breaks up the cycle, so that it proceeds in those painful bumps we call menstrual distress. Language, the way we define each other, can and does break up a smooth mental–physical rhythm into a jerky one, like a broken axle on a car. A skilful male put-down can bring on the menstrual blues. Such a disconnection can result in a woman at ovulation being quite unconscious of her desires and wishes at the menstruation a fortnight later.

One woman was locked into this contradiction by the fact that the two sides of her cycle had become strangers to each other. Her perception at the menstrual times was that her husband was no good for her, and she must leave him. Yet at ovulation she would feel the 'nest-making' instinct overcome the decisions she had made from the menstrual standpoint. She was not conscious of this; only aware of having serious rows that distressed her very much. Once she started to keep a diary of her cycle she found that these rows occurred fortnightly; her dreams showed a violent alteration too. She was able to see that her desire for individuality and freedom was expressed at her menstrual time, which gave her access to fresh possibilities; while her ovulation made her snuggle back into a marriage she was aware she was best out of. This enabled her to make the decision for freedom and a new life.

Another woman, highly-trained academically, was also very right-handed. After a series of crucial dreams that affirmed the excellence of the period and a radical alteration of attitude, she suddenly found that she was ambidextrous. The dreams included meeting an aristocratic friend who was hoarding used tampons like a treasure, of white turning to black, of A turning to Z, of the word 'transformation' written up, and of waking dreams of columns coloured black, white and red – ancient ritual colours.

There may be a rhythm in brain lateralization that accords with the menstrual rhythm, like a moon in the brain. At ovulation, which asserts left-brain qualities of coping and homemaking, it could be that the left brain is emphasized; while at the creative time of primary process, menstruation, the balance is restored towards the right brain. The woman with her easier access to both hemispheres can call on either set of abilities, depending on her interior will, and what she is educated into. Again, the emphasis in modern society is against giving both the menstrual and the right-brain qualities proper room. The original feminine unity and balance has been attacked and almost destroyed by society's left-brain emphasis.

Just as ovulation and menstruation have their individual enjoyments, so do right brain and left brain. Both ovulation and left brain have to do with *doing*, and are extrovert; both menstruation and right brain have to do with *being* and are introvert. Behaviour appropriate to either hemisphere or to either cycle culmination will facilitate access to that mode's capabilities. If you feel – in your feminine whole brain – a left-brain imbalance, then you must do right-brain things such as drawing with your left hand, or reading a good ghost story.

In left brain, the ability for abstract thought leads to abstraction and depersonalization such as one sees in modern physics, which is so out of touch with daily life and philosophy. Why does science not study the menstrual cycle thoroughly, instead of leaving it in right-brain darkness?

Too much lateral specialization is dangerous. Left brain's book is *1984*, or the emptied worlds of Pinter and Beckett, the manipulations of Burroughs or De Sade; right brain's book is romantic by, say, Rilke or Virginia Woolf. Left brain's view of right brain is the tragedy of Goethe's *Faust* Part I; right brain's view of itself is the glittering alchemical pageant of Part II.

Ovulation's view of menstruation and vice versa tore at least one great modern poet apart: in Sylvia Plath's poetry the conflict is extreme. In 'The Munich Mannequins' sexual pleasure without offspring is the ultimate selfishness; yet still 'the blood flood is the flood of love' and in 'Kindness' the blood jet is poetry.

The division between the two human modes is obviously extreme. In Christian mythology the image of woman is thus split. There is the Virgin Mary, standing for ovulation and its values, the woman who had a child without having sex; and there is the holy whore Mary Magdalen, who had sex without having a child. Our society – ferociously competitive, territorial, overweeningly visual with its conspicuous consumption and its VDUs in every home and office, in which appearances are all and subjectivity nothing, dedicated to the furious family breeding of the consumerist fantasy, and armed to the teeth with nuclear weapons at all home frontiers – is rampant ovulism.

Access to the right hand or the menstrual mode is facilitated by exercising any or all of the qualities typical of that mode. For the menstrual mode this would be a going-inwards, being still, entering symbolic actions and meditative states, learning to flow in thought and speech, cultivating the non-visual senses, becoming curious about magic or about everything feminine and individual, watching for one's intuitions and dreams, becoming interested in the lore of the night and the moon, becoming interested in 'primary process' – everything primitive, archaic, vivid, immediate, child-like, sensuous; and each and every one of these processes can be curative of functional PMS, POS and spasmodic dysmenorrhoea.

Right brain and menstrual strategies are also creative struggles. One can cultivate discriminatory skills, but the integrating inspiration comes from the right brain. Right-brain abilities become pronounced as the menstrual period approaches, and the non-visual senses increasingly enrich the visual ones. Doing the exercises described in Betty Edwards' excellent book *Drawing on the Right Side of the Brain* will not only improve one's drawing, but also any PMS or paramenstrual distress there may be.

Though the earlier view was that the verbal mode of thinking was specialized in the left hemisphere, this now appears to be incorrect. Technical or logical use of language does appear to be localized in the left hemisphere in men, but not in women. We doubt whether the connotative or imagistic or poetic use of language would be so localized in either man or woman. The poetic use of language is one of the openers of the right-brain mode. Reading powerful poetry about women's matters can ease PMS and bring on the period.

Men are looking for a synthesis of the two modes. Women are born with it. Elizabeth Sewell[3] says that there is familiar analytic logic, and there is its opponent, illogic; but their synthesis is the real human goal, and she calls it post-logic. Logic and illogic are natural enemies, but once allow them each their functions, then as with the opposing functions of ovulation and menstruation, there is a kind of mutual distillation between the two which leads to transformations which are truly alchemical.

Here is a confirmatory patchwork of quotations from some of the foremost researchers in the field:

> The female brain may be less lateralised and less tightly organised than the male brain. In male right-handers, for example, language seems to be rather rigorously segregated to the left hemisphere, while their visual-spatial skills are as rigorously segregated to the right. This does not seem to be true in right-handed females. *Their* hemispheres seem to be less functionally distinct from each other and more diffusely organised. And switching between them seems easier ... a shot of sodium amytal in one or the other of the carotid arteries ... which for a short time puts one of the hemispheres asleep ... the awake hemisphere is then given a number of language tests ... And I've found that the men and women perform quite differently. The women perform best when they have both hemispheres available, and less well when either hemisphere is out of action. The men perform best when their right hemisphere is not available, less well when both hemispheres are intact and very much more poorly – worse than the women – when their left hemisphere is out of action ... the hemispheres of men and women are differently organised ... women respond more to stimuli, generate more electricity in both verbal and visual-spatial tasks, and learn to regulate their brain-wave frequencies across the hemispheres more easily than men do ... the brains of men and women are both differentially constituted and differentially supplied with blood. When women perform verbal and visual-spatial tasks, their left and right hemispheres seem to use larger amounts of energy than men's do ... studies ... that have persistently demonstrated the abilities of females in particular areas: their superiority in certain important verbal skills; their better fine-motor co-ordination; their ability to pick up and respond to peripheral information and to read the emotional content of faces; their sensitivity to odours and their extreme sensitivity to the presence and variation of sound ... The evidence, you

see, is that the hemispheres of male brains are specialists – they speak different languages, verbal and visual-spatial. And it may be that they can communicate with each other only in a formal way, after encoding into abstract representations. The hemispheres of female brains, on the other hand, don't seem to be such specialists. And they may be able to communicate in a much less formal, less structured and more rapid way ... it's entirely possible that females are much better than males at integrating verbal and non-verbal information ... males may be at a double disadvantage in their emotional life. They may be emotionally less sophisticated. And because of the difficulty they may have in communicating between their two hemispheres, they may have restricted verbal access to their emotional world ... visual-spatial functions are lateralised in the male and more bilaterally organised in the female.[4]

Stan Gooch[5] has argued persuasively that there are deeper contradictory modes by far in the human organism, between cerebral hemispheres and the lower brain, the cerebellum, and, very important, between the two modes of the autonomic nervous system, the sympathetic and the parasympathetic. The sympathetic is the fight or flight system, the injector of adrenalin into the blood system: the parasympathetic deals with everything that is still and deep and calm. Therefore two modes are present at more than one level in the nervous system that correspond very closely to the active ovulation mode and the still menstrual mode. It is certain that the autonomic balance alters during the menstrual cycle. This double rhythm of menstruation–ovulation calls upon the whole range of opposites in the human person, psychological and physiological.

Associated with the right brain is that cast of personality sometimes called 'divergers', that is people with a markedly inventive imagination. Left-brain emphasis belongs more to 'convergers', who prefer the conventional way of thought. Ideally, everybody draws on both. If you are a diverger, you are more at home with the menstrual state, and although you will suffer some separation anxiety after ovulation (every fertile person does), you are not so likely to suffer PMS. You must beware, however, of transitional POS. You may have a lot of blood at the periods, with cramp as though the womb were trying for an orgasm. The bleeding may go on longer, as if you wanted linger there. You may feel quite nostalgic as the cycle moves on and you enter the menstrual separation.

Similarly, your sister who is a converger may be most at home in the ovulation state, may feel exalted by it, and therefore suffers separation anxiety when it is over, and terror or depression as the inventive and vivid menstrual events begin. There will be little menstrual separation anxiety, and an eager transition to ovulation, for which she is consciously prepared. Any woman will find these attitudes altering through her life, and, if she knows her cycle, will be able to account for the alterations of feelings and like or dislike of herself, and thus change through with as little distress as possible.

We quoted one study in *The Wise Wound* in particular which pointed out that the recall pattern of dreams for divergers 'is similar to that of oestrogen secretion during the menstrual cycle, and that for convergers parallels the progesterone secretion curve'.[6] The divergers may have a dream reaction to oestrogen, which helps them approach ovulation, and the convergers may have a dream reaction to progesterone, which helps them approach menstruation. Progesterone is sometimes given by injection for severe PMS such as you might find among very motherly, full-breasted, convinced 'convergers', and oestrogen for dysmenorrhoea, frequent among 'divergers' who are often dark with smaller breasts. It is a pity that no dream-records appear to have been kept in parallel with these treatments. Charting the dream-cycle would very likely decrease the necessity for hormone intervention. Any woman will find these attitudes altering through her life, and if she knows her cycle, will be able to account for the alterations of feelings and like or dislike of herself, and thus change through with as little distress as possible.

12. Beyond Logic: The Right Brain

By right-brain things we mean all those things which are significant, yet illogical. It is illogical to dress in electric blue to signify the acute energies of the pre-menstrual time, but it is significant. It is illogical to dress in red to say to oneself, 'It's come, and I'm proud of it', yet that is certainly significant, and many women do it without calculation, and may be surprised when it is pointed out. Symbolism in all its modes is the essence of shared subjective experience. A symbol is an object or act which echoes or represents a desired thing or source of energy, partakes of it, and leads one towards it. Somebody who valued the menstrual experience above the ovulation experience or any other part of the cycle, might wear a red stone at all times, and the thought of that red stone, if it was a cherished thing, would help make access to the menstrual state easier. The red stone might well be a help or companion during the difficult dreams of the premenstrual time; one might meet it initially in a dream, and then choose a stone in the actual waking world as close as possible to its kind. Many women wear lunar earrings, brooches, necklaces or rings, not only because these silver objects look good, but because, in that feeling or looking right, the cycle is being conjured into easier movement, as easy, ideally, as the moon changes. It is illogical to talk to the moon and ask the moon for advice, but it is significantly useful, and many women regard it as a companion or a friend. Ask the moon a question, and then listen inwardly for a reply. This may be the beginning of moon-synchrony.

Many women wear the Ankh or looped cross, often in silver, or the red Tat cross, the one with a double tail. Both these emblems probably represent the menstrual blood. The Tat certainly represents Isis' sanitary towel, and the Ankh too, probably, though it is abstracted to mean the Tie of Fertility, which is signed by the menstrual blood. There is a beautiful picture of Isis in the British

Museum in which she is wearing two Tat earrings which look like little men counselling into her ears. Sometimes in the menstrual state one may seem to get advice from the child that was not conceived at the earlier time of ovulation: it is the form the unconscious takes as counsellor. Again, illogical, but significant, and very helpful.

To this section belongs all creative activity. Just as the cycle should unify menstrual and ovulation states, and the brain unify its left- and right-hand modes, so creative work explores and if successful unifies these opposites.

Any loved object can hold a symbolic charge and keep it safe. One may find one's navigating signs and symbols in everyday objects which can help one over one's thresholds. On the cycle's journey one can leave signposts, cairns and caches, one is trail-blazing; in the amnesia of the changes such indicative keepsakes may seem inappropriate or even silly, and one must not throw away at ovulation the symbols of menstruation. One may even write a letter to that other person – 'Dear Red Sister...', 'Dear White Sister...' – and that would be part of a journal, which, again, would be part of the menstrual mandala.

One can communicate with that other self (and incidentally with the family too) by taking photographs in the four weeks, at the happiest time of any of the stations. Good photographs will reveal alternative personalities to an extent which is surprising. The contours of the face and expression change sometimes quite radically due to the movements of tension, mood and fluid, and this is as true of the male partner as the female.

There is an asymmetry of the face in most people, the left-hand side reflects the disposition of the right brain, and vice versa. Remember, men can get stuck in left-brain attitudes, and this can show in an expression. Woman by nature and by virtue of the cycle pass easily from mode to mode, unless a male partner's inertia detains her. This can be the wrong facial expression at an inappropriate time. By cutting up photographs one can get the look of a whole menstruous right-brain person or a whole left-brain ovulatory person, and address journal letters to that person: 'Dear White Sister, as you put on a little weight while you are ovulating, wouldn't it be best to wear separates?' 'Dear Red Sister, thank you for your concern, I think you look smashing in red.'

As Virginia Woolf knew, everybody should have a 'room of their own'. Not everybody is this lucky. If you have your own room, then it must be absolutely yours. You have the chance of using it by strengthening its atmosphere. You can do this by 'diffusing' the appropriate aromatherapy oil; by collecting objects that have a special paramenstrual significance, images of goddesses, pictures of various kinds, and perhaps a large menstrual mandala of one's own design. Others should enter only upon invitation, and that very sparingly. If you have only the workplace of the kitchen, living room or bedroom, any or all of these imply a motherly stereotype. A woman needs a non-motherly room. She needs to create a place in the home outside the stereotype. Ovulation rooms are seldom required, as the ordinary family home is an ovulation place anyway. She should furnish her menstrual room with reminders and evidence of whatever is non-motherly. This will depend on her skills, from engineering to basketweave to photography. This room might resemble a witch's cave or a high-tec lab; anything which establishes one's second self.

If no room is possible, a 'menstrual kit' is. (It can be an 'ovulation kit' for the paraovulatory time if the coming on of the ovulation has the most difficult thresholds.) It can be a cupboard or box in which all is kept pertaining to menstruation/ovulation: jewellery, clothes, tampons, sanitary towels, if one likes, a whole menstrual person. It can include make-up which can be taken out and used when the period arrives and contemplated when it is due; keepsakes of all the good things that have happened during menstrual times; red clothes, which for many people are satisfying to wear and seem actually to help the flow by that signalling and satisfaction. Some people of the Middle East and Africa have an ornamented belt which hangs on a special place on the wall; when it is not there it means the belt is in use and the woman of the house is menstruating.

Thus the change within ourselves from phase to phase is recognized and does not arrive as a mysterious, resisted attack. Men will often be glad to enjoy these signals, even to contrive some that mark their own changes in response to the cycle, or which are declarations of accord with the woman, such as a red garment, or scarf, for example.

Perfumes are not recommended as signals (though they may be in use in the bath or in evaporators or in massage as a part of aromatherapy) except very sparingly, as the natural smell of a menstruating woman is a potent means of communication: many women emit a subtle perfume that resembles a mixture of gorse (a little like coconut), opium (which is a little like chocolate) and chloroform. The pre-menstrual smell can be quite distinctive too, and it can be a warning odour resembling the discouraged sweat of a drinker, lightly alcoholic. The self-smell can feed back in PMS or POS, and that can be a good reason to try the intervention of aromatherapy.

Ideally, people and partners should enjoy their own natural smells, or find the perfume which enhances rather than swamps them. The direct smell of a tampon or sanitary towel has to be *learned* as it is too powerful for people not used to it; but when learned it carries a great deal of loving emotion. Some couples may devise a ritual of attention to the period which involves actions with the blood such as body-painting, and the blood is there for oral sex and other such full participation.

It has been said that no woman knows herself until she has tasted her menstrual blood; if true, this is a part of the menstrual affirmation. Some people find oral sex is a sovereign remedy for PMS. The male semen can be mingled with the saliva, exchanged from mouth to mouth, divided between the partners, and swallowed after long tasting. This is best done in anticipation of any bad pre-menstrual days, predicted by the menstrual mandala. The man can take juice from the vagina, and the two elixirs mingled in the mouths, or the two can be mingled in the vagina and brought up to his partner's mouth by the male. This 'white meal' needs to be taken before anxiety and hydration begins. The 'red meal' in which the mingled fluids during menstruation are exchanged in a kiss, will in certain people help dysmenorrhoea. Many hormones and prostaglandins are being exchanged and administered; but there is also a wholesome commitment and a kind of sex magic in these practices which puts energy in the cycle that passes many external and internal barriers, and enhances the sensitivities of the partners to one another in the changes of the cycle.

Menstrual rites such as these can set up a glowing desire to be *in* the period and looking forward to the period helps one to cross its thresholds.

If you are writing or tape-recording a letter to yourself at one of the culminations, listen to it at a threshold time. It is the voice of the achieved culmination of ovulation or menstruation drawing you forward over the threshold, like an initiated sister. At the threshold, the listener may not believe, but listens, and is drawn over the difficulty. The small room which you have created for yourself is the direct translation into reality of a potent dream-symbol of the passage from one state to another, a little room, sometimes joining two houses, back to back.

Thresholds are always guarded, sometimes by one's own settled prejudices, sometimes by the energies of the cycle, which may be daunting and mountainous from the hither side. The dreams often record these encounters in detailed feminine imagery that is archetypal and exclusive to the woman. So one can pass thresholds waking and sleeping.

Obviously, a book such as this cannot be all-encompassing; it is, rather, a manual of experiments. Only when women make their own experiments, believing that their cycle has actual and effective meaning, will new information be collected; many women will see it as their responsibility to spread and gather information about this subject, and to gather together to share this information. If so, please discuss the good news first, not the bad. Friends, daughters, mothers, daughter-in-laws can be talked to about periods, and maybe one will discover unexpected synchronies and sympathies. If several of you have synchronous periods you might like to meet several times a month. On menstruation day you could have a small party to celebrate. This could be the seed of an important self-help or support group which might attract other women. Talking and sharing with other women is one of the best cures for PMT or POS.

Watch how your children behave at climaxes in the cycle. Children's dreams often closely reflect the mother's cycle. Notice how *they* change during the cycle; their dreams will often be clearer than those of an adult.

It is essential to take as much sleep as possible pre-menstrually. Energy at this time – especially if it is under negotiation – can peak and then depart, leaving one in a trough. When energies are low, one must rest. Much pain comes from over-work and consequent stress at the time when a woman needs to rest and contemplate. Frantic tiring displacement activity, whatever the phase of the cycle, is a war-virtue, nothing a woman needs, and must be distinguished from genuine pre-menstrual effervescence.

Continuity in the cycle can often be established or emphasized by having a favourite walk that one takes by oneself. Please consider how it changes as you change, how the known places are familiar, but different, and how you are essentially the same person, but entering different states. You are likely to meet yourself on these walks, perhaps walking off pre-menstrual rage or using energy. You remember this, and can see differently from your present vantage-point, because that was last week and you are menstruating now. On your walk the meaning of that rage might very well emerge. Because all such rages have their meaning, one must not dismiss any of it as 'witchiness'. Acceptance of these other facets of oneself make for unification.

Galleries and museums are places designed for contemplation, and should be visited as far as possible in your most contemplative cycle-mood. Feminine images should be sought. Churches often have the right timeless atmosphere, though many women will be put off by coloured windows full of bearded patriarchs. Some prefer to contemplate the femaleness of the font, rather than the maleness of the altar. If there is a Lady Chapel, that is good to visit, but even then one should recall that orthodox Christian tradition celebrates childbirth and therefore the ovulation side of the cycle. The holocaust of wise women or 'witches' during the Renaissance was in effect a persecution of the menstrual or non-child-bearing side of the cycle – thus preventing the completion of the cycle as a whole. The Christian myth reflects this divided idea of woman: at the ovulation station stands the Virgin Mary, and at the menstruation station stands Mary Magdalen, the woman who was cured of her issue of blood and her seven devils by inadvertently brushing against Jesus' garment, and who was the first person to meet Jesus after his resurrection. Sexuality for transformation's sake is not celebrated in the Christian Church, and the image of woman is split on that issue.

Speaking of Christian imagery, there is a tradition that the Holy Ghost is feminine. One thinks of the atmosphere a woman creates, and the charged acts that a woman performs in the home during the course of her cycle; the home is not just a sanctuary but can be sacramental too, by the presence of the senior woman. Indeed, yes, churches are important places to recover one's right-brain function and one's calmness, but the feminine image has been altered by generations of male exclusivity. One might, if possible, relate to a female divine presence in church.

In gardening, menstrual blood can be used as fertilizer for bulbs, cuttings, etc. These plants are your other children. It may be thought too witch-like an involvement to feed menstrual blood to one's domestic animals, but they will surely know the period has come, and be particularly affectionate; you will want to return their love in deep menstruous tranquillity.

This is how one woman crossed that particular threshold of pain-pleasure before her period:

'For several hours, a pain, small and crampy, but very deep, from the [cervix] cone ... then tension melts, I grow excited and feel pleasure throughout my body and mind, and that comes from what was the little pain. Then, the caressing pain brings its gift, a red streak, warm and from the depths, the womb's gift, its very self, snake-skin shed again. When the first blood comes I wait as long as possible before using tampax or towel, wanting to feel the warmth and wetness of it as well as the roots of it. The pain grows heavier with the flow, like a big ache through the belly but again this is all right – it is a confirmation, a chord sung in response to the period. It lasts perhaps an hour, perhaps all day, and it feels like a companion. A new place has been made, a fresh start, a flowering.'

On the last day of her period she recorded the four days of a menstrual state that sent an afterglow through almost the whole cycle.

'This morning (not bothering now to wear a towel) one bright red gush of blood – farewell. All the days of the bleeding, great ease and calmness of mind, powerful sexual feeling, big elaborate orgasms both from clitoris and thrusting sex combination of the whole. Immense interest in the forms of the world, skies, trees, houses, people. Richness of existence re-revealed by the period, and, this being so, this high plateau of feeling will probably last until the week before the next period. Then a low, bad-tempered time usually comes.'

Even though she had found her treasure at that time in the period itself, there was still a difficult threshold to be negotiated at the end of the pre-menstrual week, at the pre-menstrual transition. Perhaps it can be seen as the change-over from the luteal hormones of the ovary to the action of womb-secretions at the period. From ovulation's side that 'small, crampy pain' would feel like a depressing barrier, the period treasure guarded by a nipping serpent. Then, once accepted, the pain led her into the treasure-chamber again.

13. The Two Cycles

To go with the two human modes, there are not just the two culminations of one cycle, menstruation and ovulation, but actually two cycles, one belonging to the ovaries and one to the womb. This mirror-imaging resembles brain lateralization.

The sequence for the ovary starts on the first day of menstruation and lasts an average of twenty-eight days. The first stage, called the follicular stage, is the development of the Graafian follicle. This follicle consists of the ovum in its 'storage' state, surrounded by nutritive cells which, as the follicle ripens, secrete oestrogen. It drills its way to the surface of the ovary. In due course it ruptures and releases the egg, which floats into the Fallopian tube. This will be at roughly Day 12 to 17 of a twenty-eight-day cycle. The burst follicle stays on the surface of the ovary and, influenced by pituitary hormones, gets a new lease of life as the corpus luteum, the producer of progesterone, the hormone which prepares the womb-wall for implantation. If the ovum is not fertilized, this corpus luteum begins to regress ten days after it began to develop. Its full life-span is fifteen days, which explains why menstruation fairly regularly occurs fifteen days after ovulation. Eventually the corpus luteum disappears, leaving a small white scar. The surface of the ovary is pitted with these scars like the surface of the moon.

The climax of the ovarian cycle, quite naturally, is ovulation. It is the womb-cycle which is properly called the menstrual (or endometrial) cycle. The lining of the womb acts as a kind of mirror to the ovarian events, though there is now evidence of feed-back from the womb itself by means of prostaglandin and other mechanisms. The whole makes a very complex system, because there is undoubtedly feed-back from the womb to the brain's hypothalamus to the pituitary to the ovary to the womb; but every system in the body is immersed in the actions of every other system. The womb has its clocks too.

THE TWO CYCLES

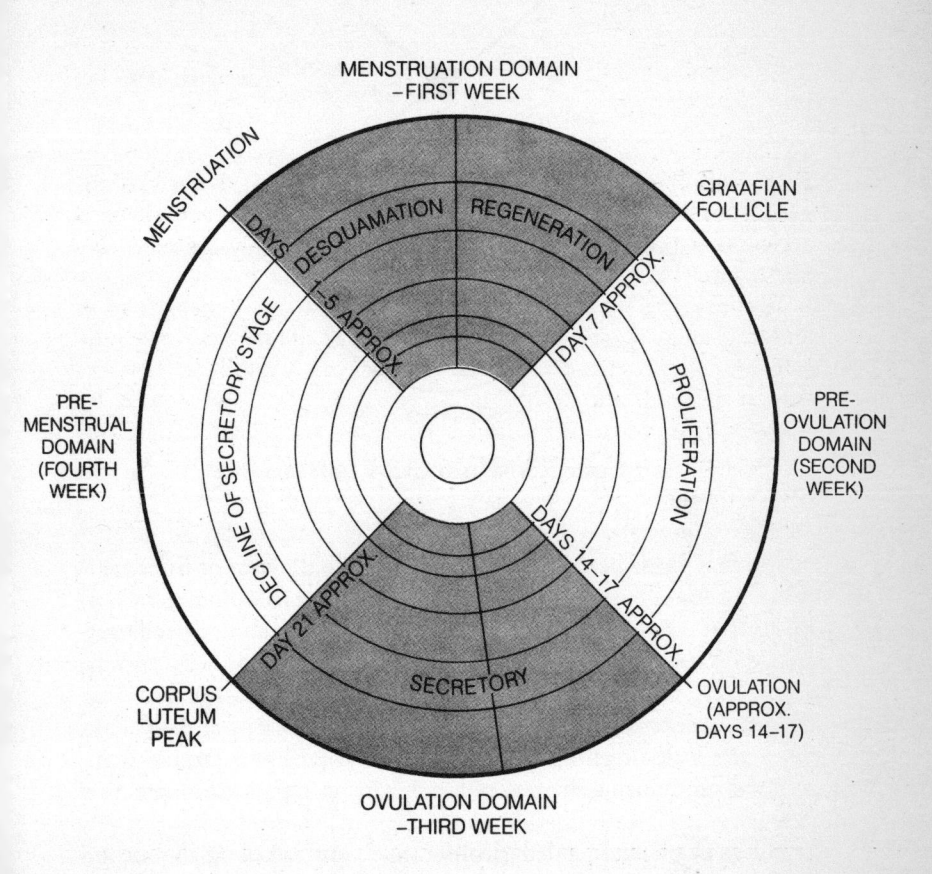

Figure 4. *Combined Menstrual and Ovarian Cycles*
Two cycles – the menstrual and the ovarian, each with different potentialities in interplay – combine to express the female rhythm.

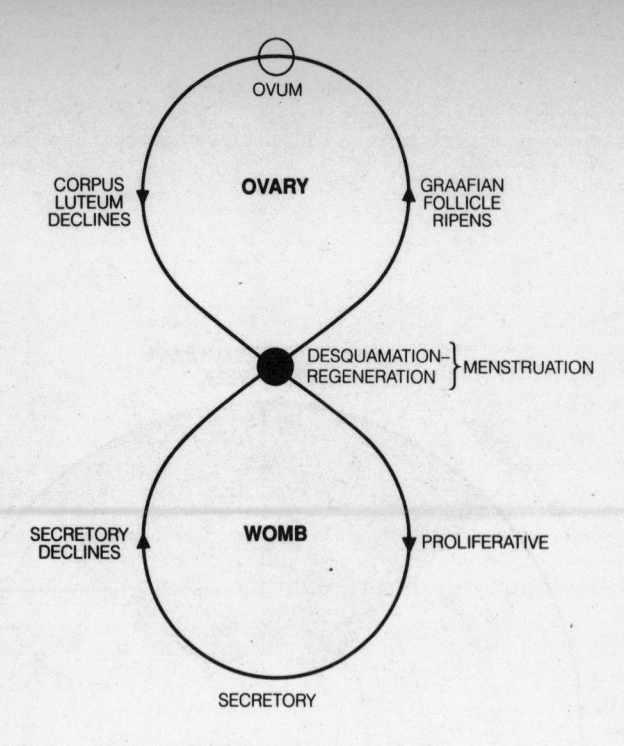

```
                    OVUM
        CORPUS              GRAAFIAN
        LUTEUM    OVARY     FOLLICLE
        DECLINES            RIPENS

                 DESQUAMATION–  ⎫
                 REGENERATION   ⎬ MENSTRUATION
                                ⎭

        SECRETORY   WOMB    PROLIFERATIVE
        DECLINES

                  SECRETORY
```

Figure 5. *The Two Cycles Unfolded*

The first phase of the menstrual cycle – usually four or five days – is the shedding of the womb-wall. The traditional ovulatory view of this is that the 'uterus weeps in memory of the ovum departed fourteen days previously', while the menstrual view may very well be 'Phew! rest, creativity and peace at last!' The second stage makes up the first week; this is the regenerative phase of about three days when the inside of the womb, which has been like a large raw interior wound during the first phase, begins to repair itself with new cells.

The next phase is called 'proliferative', and takes up the second week, coming to a close at ovulation. Under the influence of oestrogen poured out from the ripening follicle in the ovum the womb-lining thickens and vascularizes. This can be regarded as nest-building or home-building. In the proliferative phase it is as though the foundations and walls of the home are being put in, as well as the plumbing. The next phase is called the 'secretory' phase, and this is as though the larder is being stocked – the womb-lining prepares for possible fertilization by producing secretions that can

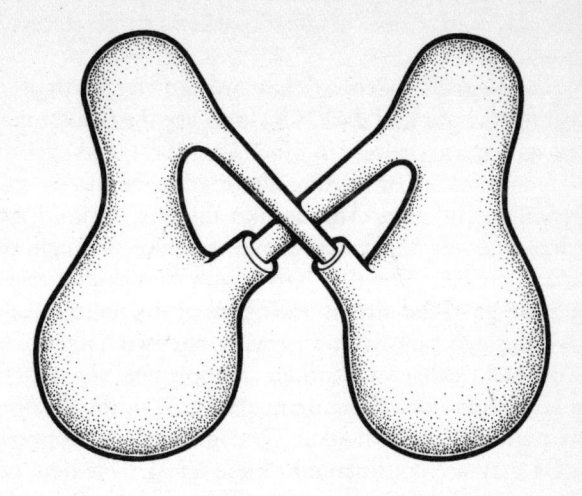

Figure 6. *The Double Pelican*

nourish the ovum. This happens under the influence of progesterone, at ovulation. If there is no fertilization, the corpus luteum begins to shrink and on the last day of the cycle menstruation becomes imminent, and this, failing pregnancy, is the big womb event.

It is usual to superimpose the two cycles, as in the convenient and symbolic moon cycle we started with, two culminations and two thresholds. It is interesting to note that the moon cycle was originally depicted by the famous Chinese sign of the Yin-Yang, of balancing dynamic opposites. In the case of the feminine cycle, when the corpus luteum is exhausted, the menstruation begins to appear, and after the ovum is shed the womb begins to wax, the egg to wane. As soon as one process ends, the other begins. When the moon is full, blackness begins to appear on its surface, and only when it is dark does the light begin to appear again. The Yin-Yang sign was originally a moon-calendar, and is basic to the most ancient book in the world, the *I Ching*, a weather and earth oracle.

One can unfold the two cycles into their interlocking components to make a figure-8, the mathematical sign for infinity. The Trumps of the Tarot – another oracle based on intuition or right-brain perception – in many systems are laid out in a figure-8. It is sometimes useful to play with these 'magical' patterns to get access to right-brain qualities.

The moon–earth system snakes around the earth in a spiral, intertwining its light and dark. One may see the menstrual–ovarian cycle too as a spiral process in time. Any of these images may be of assistance in thinking or musing about your menstrual mandala as it stretches out in time. This is like the Yin-Yang stretched out concertina-wise, or the wheel-cross spinning through time with other wheel-crosses. The two halves may be distilled together, enriching both, as in the alchemical figure of the double pelican; and the Yin-Yang sign can show, as it were, the two halves of the brain enriching each other with their complementary functions, or heaven and earth interchanging qualities, as in the *I Ching*.

Many patterns can be made by the interaction of opposites, and as we said they are considered to be magical. This may not be entirely coincidental if one believes that the mind produces *symbols* of things that are tabooed, or holy, or too large for the individual, or that are unnoticed but all-pervasive, such as the dual menstrual rhythm. Symbols are ways of getting in touch with unconscious knowledge.

14. Rites of Passage

We have already mentioned how the placebo effect can be seen as a symbolic gesture which acts powerfully on the psyche. Modern life has too few of these symbolic acts, which are sometimes called rites of passage,[1] as they enable the person using or undergoing them to pass from one mental, social or physical state to another. The term is usually used for transition or transformations from one stage of life to another, for example from infancy to puberty or puberty to adulthood, and in some societies there are ceremonies which mark the menarche or first menstruation of the woman. The rites of passage of menarche define the new resources that a woman will find in herself, and they do that by a ceremony in which symbolic actions carry the information; alternatively, it is directly given by a wise woman initiator. Information will be appropriate to the new situation of menstruator and mother. In the West we have no such ceremonies which help the child adapt to her new status as woman, or which make the changes she is experiencing friendly; this is an index of the neglect of the menstrual cycle in our culture.

Just as there are rites of passage from puberty to adulthood, and these are not developed in our world, so there are rites of passage within the menstrual cycle which can be recovered by the individual out of her dynamically-active unconscious personality, and used for her benefit.

Usually, rites of passage are subdivided into rites of separation, transition rites, and rites of incorporation. We will see that dreaming is a process of discovering images of these changes. A person may separate from ovulation-feelings with a lurch, wanting a new child, to a transition time when everything is in flux, followed by reincorporation as a person capable of menstruation. When this natural cyclical process is followed in dream-life, there will be found there the symbols of separation from ovulation and entry to menstruation, and these 'visions of the night' ease the passage from the one state to the next. Any strategy which we suggest you adopt in these pages is a rite of passage, following the rule that anything which moves energy round the cycle works against distress. Even meeting a friend whose period has 'come on' can be like a greeting that eases one's own period or its anticipations.

Becoming aware of these rhythms in oneself, one becomes aware of them in nature. Most of us neglect direct participation in natural rhythms, of the weather, of the moon, of the sun and the seasons. We have failed to develop our sense of how energy oscillates in the body and outside. Becoming initiated into one's menstrual rhythms is an initiation into further sensitivities to the natural world. These sensitivities and their meaning for the individual lie mainly in the neglected aspect of the cycle, the menstrual bleeding itself. No wonder it is a difficult initiation, as women's processes are at the fringe of our culture, and resisted by those at the controlling centre, which favours ovulation.

The menstrual distress we experience (too often blindly, physically, without imagery) is the involuntary *initiation*, composed of the worry and pain of *separation*, the new feelings and knowledge of *transition*, the adjustments of *reincorporation*. PMS, the main problem, is the *separation* from ovulatory values, the *transition* into menstrual values, and *reincorporation* into their new values. The menstrual role is the least known and least favoured in our society, and this is why PMS is so widespread. It is the stirring of a new womanhood. Spasmodic dysmenorrhoea (painful period bleeding) has to do with the reincorporation into the menstrual world; the womb has new work, not child-bearing, to perform. It is significant that spasmodic dysmenorrhoea responds well to the same techniques used in natural childbirth, or to an orgasm.

Pre-ovulatory distress is the initiation into the ovulatory role, well understood and over-emphasized in most women, which is why it is not so frequent as PMS. However, it is frequent in women who are uncertain whether or not they should have or want children, and particularly evident in women who have decided that they will not have children, and have been sterilized, perhaps with tubal ligation. Then the approach to ovulation may be their most sensitive time, and PMS is rare if they have decided to side with the menstrual culmination.

15. A Useful Waking-dream Technique

Difficult transitions can be helped by various waking-dream techniques. You could term this one 'calling each other down'. It goes with a cuddle, preferably naked, or after sex; it is a way of using that state of hypnotic openness of floating in and out of sleep, which can be charged with images mutually exchanged and changing.

The first one to see images tells the partner who, if she/he is 'floating', will see them too, altered. Each tells the other, in a kind of mutual feed-back hypnosis. The images alter, blend, interact, and open out new vistas. Images can be used from poetry, from sci-fi, from your own dreams, or from anywhere else where a captivating image calls for you, such as from time spent together.

This kind of work has been quite extensively explored in drug states, but drugs are not necessary at all. Each partner can accept this hypnotic communion, for that is what it is, and allow the other to soothe him/her into greater relaxations than either can manage alone. The recounting partner keeps a hold on consciousness while the other listens, goes deeper and then takes over. Eventually no voices are needed, and you float away, perhaps into the same dream.

'Calling each other down', is analogous to the 'staircase' of deepening climaxes during sex when both man and woman hold on to consciousness a little longer each time to increase the other's pleasure as it rises to mutual and irresistible orgasm. It is also similar to the hypnotist's rapport, but with a trusted partner. Couples who practise this kind of communication and become used to rapport of this kind will find their best abilities open up to them. A kind of incipient dreaming goes on in people all the time, but, 'the point is that the dream should not be interpreted in terms of ordinary reality, but rather, this reality in terms of the dream'.[1]

ONE: *'Feel sun on your face. Open your inner eyes. We're gardening. There's an old stone well coping in the middle of the lawn. Help me slide the lid off.'*

THE OTHER: *'As the lid slides off I lean quite safely and see the gleam of water far below, smell stone and water in the draught of air that blows up at us. Bird-song seems to be coming from far below. There are steps spiralling down. Will you go first or shall I? I'll get the torches.'*

ONE: *'I'll go first. It's quite safe. The stairs are flat long slabs of stone. There's a rail to hold on to. At last I'm at water-level. There's a circular ledge all round, like a path. I can see a passage straight ahead. Let me help you down. Now we're walking along the passage.'*

THE OTHER: *'At the end of the passage is an immense chamber in the rock. Our torch-beams fade away in its immensity. It echoes with water-sounds. There is water here, all around.'*

ONE: *'Let's shut the torches off and let our eyes get accustomed to the dark. There's a house standing on an island in the lake's centre.'*

THE OTHER: *'There are tall trees on the island as well as the house. I can hear the murmuring of water. The lake is moving.'*

ONE: *'The lake is revolving round and round the island. The air is cool and fresh, I can hear it in the trees. The walls of the chamber are shining very gently. The house stands on the cone of the island.'*

THE OTHER: *'The windows are lighting up, as if somebody with a taper were going from room to room lighting candles.'*

ONE: *'There's a rowing boat this side of the lake. You can hardly see it at first, it's painted twilight-colour. Let's get in, row across and knock at the door.'*

THE OTHER: *'And ask to see the well.'*

ONE: *'The house will have a well.'*

THE OTHER: *'And when we have met the one who lives there perhaps we can enter it.'*

ONE: *'The light from the opening door strikes across the water like a broad path.'*

Though the visual sense is used in this co-guided imagery tour it is supported by non-visual images of smell, touch and movement. In fact, whenever the flow of visualization checks, it is good policy to search inwardly for a non-visual sensation, which will start it going again, as it is the non-visual which has the better access to creative right-brain modes.

This kind of exercise is a going-within, a sinking-down, which is why it is usual to find that female images occur spontaneously. One can of course direct one's visualizations into, say, the peaks of mountains; but when in relaxation the images are allowed simply to pop into the head, they most often lead downwards, to female regions. Taking a left-hand pathway downwards may lead one too quickly into right- or lower-brain regions. It is best to travel to one's right at first. Sometimes it is useful to break through a floor or ground-layer, when further subterranean layers, often lighted, may be found and explored. With practice, the result is a kind of lucid or waking dream.

By going down one can tap the water-table of these images, so neglected in our culture; their occurrence and presence will assist transitions. Each new 'calling down' can start with a spontaneous image of relaxation, or it can start at some fruitful point in the previous co-guided imagery: for example, who answered the door of the house on the island? Perhaps they did, or the child they had not had.

If frightening images occur, they can be transformed by the other partner's caress, if one is truly relaxed. One can become that frightening image and look out from its eyes, but that is better done fully waking.

A high degree of rapport can come through relaxation exercises, the Eeman circuit, sexual exploration and dream-sharing. One can start by requesting an image or a situation to do with the period. One woman during her period was told to visualize being in a place that symbolized her period. She found herself in a green meadow which contained a round area marked in quadrants, ready for her to travel through successively. There was an area of water, a tunnel, an area of fire, and an area of mountains. She chose to travel in the mountains, and there met a 'dishy' and angelic young man who gave her advice. This experience led her to further dream-work which completely altered her experience of her cycle and relocated a troublesome third week's distress to slight irritability at pre-ovulation. (It is worth noting that the Celtic purgatory was imaged as four fields.)

The co-guided imagery tour quoted above would probably be

during late pre-menstrual transition, the light in the house then would be the blood beginning, and the person in the house a helpful feminine figure of knowledge and power. Your partner in this co-guided tour, if male, would have to pass muster with this figure, or perhaps claim affinity with a male figure also living harmoniously in this house. The cone in the cavern, or the cone-shaped hill with a grove of trees on it – the omphalos or cervix-cone – is an ancient and frequent symbol which powerfully aids transitions.

The putting-on of various clothes, with their patterns of colours, openings and perfumes, and their shaped caress, is a form of shared imagery. A man should be accustomed to the feeling of his clothes on his skin, not as an assertion of 'power over' but of power within. Men's clothes are so often adapted to convey a macho image. Impulses to wear loose-fitting clothes that do not delineate various areas of the body should be explored; comfortable unisex clothes, for instance; 'anima clothes', colourful and scented; dreaming clothes.

Frightening images during relaxation exercises and guided imagery of waking dreams often appear safely 'distanced'. Whereas in a pre-menstrual dream one may be threatened with decapitation, in a relaxation imagery-tour one may merely *find* a head on a platter. Neglected energies in the womb are frequently symbolized by a severed head with prophetic powers, sometimes by the angel Lucifer dropped head-first from heaven with hair incandescent from re-entry, like a meteorite. Death and resurrection imagery, and therefore life-in-death imagery, is a feature of the cycle-transitions and separation. The imagery is the first expression in dreams, and ignorance of the meaning creates fear, which creates nightmares, which, suppressed, cause distress in the transitions. This is why we can diminish PMS and other distress by dreaming into these events. One becomes accustomed to one's personal narrative that dovetails with them, and learns something of the collective narrative, which, as it is of the woman, is exiled and called paganism.

The woman religion is deeply involved with this integration of the cycle; the cycle is the narrator, and the religious images are the narrative of the cycle. No wonder there is so much PMS, with little of this deep and potentially religious imagery of the woman properly accredited, and when its effect is safe-passing through these important states of being. The practical way of meeting the unconscious mind as expressed in the cycle is denied to people by patriarchal religion. The male spirit also appears in cycle dreams and visualizations, but divided, as the cycle is divided into ovulation and menstruation. Male influence can appear as an ovulation animus (social animal and patriarch) and a menstruation animus (human-animal-matriarchal). Part of one's task is not to be possessed by these figures, but to relate to them. It is important to realize that, even when they appear in an unpleasant form, the very look and action of animus-figures is a clue to what established masculinity has stolen from the dreamer's personality. The emblematic figure has now come to restore it, marked, as it were, and formed by his crime. The purpose is always restoration, and if these figures are ambiguous, that is part of the labyrinth one has to tread. They may appear in a positive form, and then they come with some gift of consciousness concerning what one is accustomed to call one's masculine side, which is nevertheless part of the whole person. A positive animus may change during the cycle to a threatening figure, as for instance where a kind, powerful and competent husband-figure presides over ovulation-dreams, but seems to lay blame if the egg is not fertilized, and turns angry or reproachful. This might happen during ovulation-separation, that perilous time when the egg dies and the body can seem to mourn. It is likely in most relationships that projection of these figures will take place on to the male partner. The partner may react by accepting the projection, consciously or unconsciously, and *becoming* the ideal husband (ovulation) or the sinister lover (menstruation) – or reacting completely contrary to this. Contrariness or an inability to alter response to a projected figure causes trouble when flexibility or change is needed, as with all cycle-events. Conscious and yet spontaneous play, like a dream or image-fantasy, is needed by both partners. To project unconsciously on one's partner is to be in the power of that image. Dreaming it is to relate to it, to possess and not be possessed.

One of the titles of the ancient goddess was Life-in-Death and Death-in-Life. This referred primarily to the cycles of 'death' and 'resurrection' in the personal cycle, then to the cycle of the moon and the seasons, then to the life-cycle of the person, with its promise of after-life, in a mounting series of felt knowledge. The foundation pattern for this was clear knowledge of the menstrual cycle.

Sometimes people find their own menstrual mandala, made in waking life, appearing in dreams as a guiding pattern there too – as the Round Table, for instance, or inlaid on a floor as a dancing labyrinth, or fastened together and building a great tree, of which the individual months are slices. One may perhaps taste the apple of that tree.

16. Yoga and its Analogues

Statistics show that women who exercise suffer far less from menstrual troubles than those who do not. But competitive exercise can lead to nervous strain, and it is best to adopt an activity that also has an acknowledged mental side to it. The various kinds of yoga work specifically to *yoke* mind and body – this is the meaning of the word *yoga*. Yoga's purpose is to know the body and its feelings, and to open the body's sense of itself to itself; that is also the purpose of understanding the menstrual cycle. Simply knowing the menstrual cycle is a kind of yoga, and will in itself relieve distress.

With or without yoga, regular practice of an easy relaxation technique works wonders. The one we suggest on pages 151–3 works well if practised every day, starting as the period finishes, and then going on right round the cycle. Such a practice can bring on that special feeling of increased access to a roomy, untroubled space inside. Some people find the closest analogy is the post-coital state or the menstrual state itself. Much of the periodical trouble may vanish even in the first month. Dream-recall is also improved, and one can even learn deliberately to re-dream during the relaxed state to find out what happens next. One simply calls them up before the inner eye and allows them to proceed on their own.

'Meditation' is a word that has been spoiled by religious wars, rather as the word 'menstruation' has been tainted with sexual politics. A good rule about these meditative practices is: if it didn't happen to you like this once as a child, then it is false. One is re-linking oneself to childhood experiences when a single flower was precious; when the flicker of snowfall over a darkening garden was more absorbing than any television programme. It is of such experiences of harmony that the menstrual state is made, and to which the woman is by an integrated cycle more attuned than her male partner. It is, if you like, a right-brain or whole-brain state in which 'one thought fills immensity' in its natural processes and associations, so that one dwells easily in it and then is able simply to let it go, leaving a living and restful emptiness; the outer world now energized by one's inner life.

The postures in yoga lead towards an experience of breathing that is as peaceful and rhythmical as a baby's. Most yoga books recommend special postures for increasing the health of the woman's pelvic region and therefore of the menstrual cycle – relieving congestion and spasm. But the pelvic basin is only a part of the person; the tone of the whole body improves with yoga, and this of course will also improve menstrual troubles. It is now understood that every bodily action and function releases active hormones and neuro-transmitters into the tissues and bloodstream. Thus the lungs, just as the womb does, secrete certain prostaglandins and pheromones, which emerge in the breath and are rebreathed in a mixture with similar emanations from the skin to react in a general chemical feed-back system; meanwhile, the action of yoga breathing will massage the womb itself, the ovaries, Fallopian tubes, kidneys and surprarenals, every tissue uttering its chemical note to make up a symphony of personality.

The pattern of breathing is four-fold, like the menstrual cycle itself: inhalation, hold, exhalation, hold, and each subdivision of the breathing has a special feeling. 'External retention' – when the lungs are left after exhalation to find their own moment of inhalation – corresponds in a way to the menstrual state like an emptied, creative moment.

We would like to find room to give detailed instructions, but there are many excellent books, some specifically for women. Many towns have yoga groups, and some are run by women; a yoga group may easily give rise to a self-help group in which all women's matters are discussed; and this can be the best thing of all, since meeting together can synchronize periods and adjust distress so it is minimized in the cycle, especially when dreams are shared and menstrual diaries kept. This is the true woman's yoga.

In aromatherapy the meditation trigger is the essential oil; it is easy and natural to pause within the feeling of a potent smell, and that is 'meditation'. Incense is a similar device. The simple feeling of the passage of breath through the nostrils in 'alternate nostril breathing' can so concentrate one's attention that the whole self opens out within the action, and when the actions ceases.

The flower of yoga is, however, the sexual act. The concentration on the sensations in the body is so intense that the orgasm releases the whole body with the mind into the deepest meditation and reverie possible. Many people will seek the physical release alone and simply drift in and out of the new-body feeling, grazing as it were on the day's events. The reverie can, however, be directed.

Many women find that their sexual feeling increases at both ovulation and at menstruation. It is very important that a man should be sensitive to this aspect of the cycle. Ovulation sex has its special flavour, as does menstruation, and the transition from one to the other will be eased, as the qualities in each are distinguished.

It is easy in sex to meditate on the feeling of one's own and the other's skin – that is the dark sense, of touch; to taste one's partner; and to meditate on your mutual incense; and to sink post-coitally into dream and out of it, passing thresholds of awareness in the same manner as one passes the thresholds of the cycle.

Gardening is also a yoga and a meditation; and there is nothing better to give both exercise and time itself a changed quality, especially at difficult stages of the cycle. Gardening – closeness to earth and its working – helps pass the menstrual thresholds, though one ought to start before actual distress. It is no use digging up the garden if one has menstrual cramps!

Holding and caressing a loved animal will soothe. It is a yoga, re-yoking oneself to the animal powers. When a domestic animal enters the room, the human blood-pressure goes down. When an animal such as a cat sits on your lap, there is a mutual exchange of nervous energy. Again, time alters: a threshold to a different time is passed, just as in the cycle itself. Time spent with an animal is not the same as human time. An animal can be a kind of menstrual therapist, just as it can be a mediator of menstrual and ovulatory energies in a dream, where the cat, or the dog, 'knows the way'.

Cooking too alters time, and taste is an inward sense that is emphasized menstrually. Dwelling on it can lead to an eased transition to the menstrual state. In that state the mere taste of a glass of pure water can echo and re-echo through the psyche.

Menstrual Yoga

There are two postures which are sexually differentiated in Hatha Yoga. These are the Headstand, known as the King Posture, and the Shoulderstand called the Queen Posture. The headstand is said to stimulate the cerebral hemispheres, the shoulderstand to increase circulation to the old-brain. For proper balance, men should concentrate more on the shoulderstand, and women on the headstand. This assumes that men need to be got into touch with archaic and old-brain matters, and women to the lofty abstract propositions and logic of the new brain. It is certainly good to balance these postures, though the headstand is usually regarded as difficult, and should be learned from a teacher. It is a very exhilarating posture.

People practised at yoga may like to try emphasizing headstand as they approach ovulation and shoulderstand as they approach menstruation. Watch the flow of thought in headstand – certainly it seems to formulate itself more in concepts than images; conversely, in the shoulderstand, images and body-feelings seem to predominate. Everybody knows how difficult it is mentally to move between these two modes, how difficult it is to put one's non-verbal images into words, for example, to explain something. Words used in this way are a left-brain function, denotative. If words are used for their own images and for their associations in the way of poetry, they are connotative, and draw upon the neglected right-brain's verbal abilities. Improvisation can help balance right and left brains: a songwriter will use the left brain for the words, and the right brain for the music. The two separated functions become a unity. You don't need to be a songwriter to know this! A man tends to laugh when he sees three women talking at once. 'How can they listen to each other?' he asks. But women can both talk and listen at once in complex whole-brain interactions.

There is another rhythm which may be related to left brain and right brain, alternating their functions, and this is the shrinking and swelling of the nasal tissue. Air flows predominantly through one or other at about two-hourly intervals. This rhythm can change through emotional upsets or through menstrual distress, and can be restored (eventually unified so there is an equal flow between both nostrils) by the kind of yoga-breathing which is called 'alternate nostril breathing'. The nasal and sexual engorgements are closely related, and menstrual cramps may go with a stuffiness of nose. There is a PMS condition sometimes known as 'vacuum headache' which is due to the swelling of tissues at the entrance of the nasal sinuses. Alternate nostril breathing can prevent this quite speedily, and for best results one should do it daily. If your left nostril is stuffed up, lie down on your right side for a few minutes, and relax.

The nostril should free itself, unless you have a cold coming. There is also a spot at the base of the skull which will free the nostril if it is pressed firmly.

It is very interesting in that you can actually *see* the restoration of brain-balance by practising alternate nostril breathing in front of a familiar object, a favourite painting, for example, which has grown stale with much familiarity. As you breathe you will find that the colours freshen and the perspectives deepen, and this effect signals the passing of a mild depression. One can try balancing mood too – the cross-over applies to the nostrils, and one can use the digital manipulation of nostril breathing to stimulate, say, the right brain by drawing in through the left nostril (exhaling through both). For that matter, one can do this by turning down one's stereo headphones on the right ear so as to give more volume to the left. Covering the eyes will do this also as there is a cross-over on the eyes, but it is not complete, and the fields merge. Look at the changes of mood of a picture according to whether you look at it with left or right eye! You can apply similar technique to massage, and slightly emphasize massage on the right side as an aid to passing the threshold of ovulation, which prefers left-brain pattern; and on the left side in passing through PMS to the menstrual state.

The exercises used to strengthen the pelvic floor after childbirth by internally pulling up the anus and vagina as far as they will go to the navel, trying to get them to meet, are also important – called in Chinese yoga the Deer and in Hindu *Asvini Mudra*. You wag the tail. This exercise in women should help menstrual cramps and pelvic congestion; in men it will stimulate the prostate and increase control of ejaculation. As with nostrils, ears or eyes, one can balance the body through anal contractions. It is a kind of internal massage. If you try you will find that the anus-muscles contract in a quadrant: forwards, backwards, to the left and to the right. If you want to stimulate the right brain (and all the organs on the left-hand of the body) contract the left anus more than the other three quadrants. To prepare for menstrual flow, emphasize the central part of the anus. This practice also helps the vaginal muscles and vaginal sensitivity.

As we remarked before, an orgasm, whether self-induced or with a partner, is a great aid in dysmenorrhoea, and will also help PMS and POS, providing love-making takes place well before distress is established. The orgasm will, if complete, balance the whole body.

Another exercise which opens up new dimensions in both the inner and outer world is conscious whole-breathing. One should get instructions on *pranayama* from a good yoga book, but basically whole breathing is filling and emptying, with easy continued breathing, the whole capacity of the lungs: lower abdomen, midriff and upper chest.

All forms of yoga will increase consciousness of weather sensitivity. Variations of air-pressure and electrical tension, humidity and temperature, all have their effect on the body, and if one is paying attention to movement and breathing, that effect will be quite evident, and a thing to be worked with, or around. If, as we recommend, you keep a weather-chart with the menstrual mandala, it becomes possible to predict local weather with a fair amount of accuracy. This is better far than suffering unconsciously from weather-sensitivity.

Sex Yoga

The great principle is to make love in accord with the cycle's highs and lows. Using the menstrual mandala, sexually active people, if they didn't know already, will soon find out that their sexual energy is not diffused throughout the cycle so much as concentrated at certain recurrent high spots. It is common for the most intense of these to occur at or round about the two cycle culminations: ovulation and menstruation. There may be quite strong subsidiary peaks during the receding of menstruation, at about Days 6 to 7, and, if one is lucky, during the pre-menstrual week. The luck here is that the extra energy of PM time, which in so many people turns into PMS, can have instead this strong, even riotous, sexual channel. The energy can then be shared with one's male partner instead of burning holes in the carpet, so to speak, and sex at this time can be very energizing for him, and it can bring on the period too. Sex indeed is one of the prime movers-on of the cycle, remembering the rule *Anything cures which releases energy to flow through the cycle.*

Again, we are not just bodily creatures. When you make love, you make love to mind and brain too. In physiological terms, orgasm can shift brain function from left brain to right.[1] This means that it is the gateway not only to intense physical pleasure, but also to the riches of creativity. Therefore the 'quiet time' or stillness after sex needs to be guarded. All visions, dreams and fantasies occurring sexually should be treasured, recorded and expressed. Men can understand some of the depth of that menstrual state through the orgasm, and through menstrual sex. The reverie after sex, and the reverie of the menstrual state, are closely related.

This is all quite in accord with scientific information. The neurophysiologist James Prescott, for example, in writing about the possible evolution of the species, sees a link between female sexuality and religious experience: 'unique connections between the female forebrain and cerebellum may account for the fact that some women experience orgasm so intensely that they enter altered states of consciousness similar to religious experiences.' He is despondent about men, however: 'Lacking the neurological capability to integrate pleasure into the neocortex, or higher brain centre, however, males cannot reach the same transcendent heights ... Their pleasure is largely reflexive.' He is of course speaking of left-brain man.[2]

The unique advantage human women have over all animals is menstruation. It is an evolutionary advance, since social bonding and organization can be attributed to it, as well as mental and emotional development. Prescott puts this into scientific terms: 'the sexual receptivity of most female mammals is under ovarian control ... the human sexual receptivity is not bound by ovarian cycles.' Prescott believes that sexual receptivity at times other than ovulation, as in the human female, has the primary function not of reproduction 'but the development and maintenance of affectional bonding'. He says that human males do not appear to have undergone this evolutionary change. We would say 'Maybe not yet, not all men'.

Prescott then affirms: 'this dramatic shift in the function of sexuality ... will ultimately lead towards the integration of the conscious and the unconscious mind and to a more profound understanding of the spiritual nature of the species.' Evolution gave the human female the neurobiological advantage, he maintains, so she has the essential role. 'The male will sort of tag along,' as he puts it. We are sure he can do more than this.

This view of sexuality seems then to be fairly well established scientifically. It has its historical dimensions too. According to the learned feminist writer Barbara G. Walker, this evolutionary secret has long been practised, and is a chief gift that women bring through their menstruation. She speaks of the spiritual enlightenment through sexual intercourse she calls *horasis*, and particularly the power of the 'red juice' of menstruation in giving sexual enlightenment to men.[3]

There is an interesting sidelight on this in Jan Morris's *Conundrum*. Morris, like a modern-day Tiresias, has been both sexes. She started as a man, a trans-sexual, possessed by the feeling that he was actually a woman who by some mistake had got into a man's body. This is not the place to discuss trans-sexualism generally, but Morris's description is relevant here. At the beginning of the sex change, he took female hormones for some eight years. The first effect was to rejuvenate him on the way to his goal of womanhood.

> The first result was not exactly a feminisation of my body, but a stripping away of the rough hide in which the male person is clad. I do not mean merely the body hair, nor even the leatheriness of the skin, nor all the hard protrusion of muscle: all those indeed vanished over the next few years, but there went with them something less tangible too, which I know now to be specifically masculine – a kind of unseen layer of accumulated resilience, which provides a shield for the male of the species, but at the same time deadens the sensations of the body. It is as though some protective substance has been sprayed on to a man from a divine aerosol, so that he is less immediately in contact with the air and the sun, more powerfully compacted within his own resources.

Later, after the sex-change, Jan Morris declares she entered a different world of feeling and sensation; every detail of the mundane world had been transformed, so that ordinary life became infinitely interesting.

It is only in exceptional circumstances that a man has to go so far as to *become* a woman. We are certainly not recommending 'the operation'! What we are saying is that men must be prepared to accept a certain 'feminization'. Jung says that the characteristic of the masculine is *perfection*, that of the feminine *completeness*. The habit of narrow specialization in men has to be given up, both mentally and sensuously. In ordinary everyday life (the crucible of PMS and POS) the masculine habit of either–or logic should not be given special prizes. Yeats praised the friends who did not converse as a man did, by contradictory process, but talked with one as a woman would, by extending and improvising on the other's thought. Or as Jung said, a woman gives the Object a chance.

Some men regard sex as a conquest to be enjoyed in the relaxation after relieving the sexual tension. Most people feel there is something more than the physical to be expected of sex, or more than we ordinarily think of as physical. When 'afterglow' and 'falling in love' happen, they are right-brain states, so they suffer the unfortunate repression suffered, as it were, both by the right brain and the menstrual state. You could say that good sex and menstruation are equally tabooed. It comes as no surprise then that the best sex can be had at menstruation, precisely when it is tabooed by the major religions. It is also the 'safest' time. Many scientific papers have been written denying the sexual peak that most women feel during the period, because the theory was that it could not aid survival of the species, and was therefore 'non-adaptive', and didn't exist. Science, as a left-brain activity, disregards feelings and is suspicious of creative imagination, so it cannot see that sexual intercourse in itself is 'adaptive' and does favour the survival of the species simply because it stimulates people's mentalities. It is also conveniently forgotten in most studies of dreams that they are a product of or accompanied by sexual excitement. During dreaming men and women are always sexually aroused.

The cultivation of mentality by sexuality has remained a rarity, except among women. A woman by nature is usually multi-orgasmic. The male may be jealous of this and probably can't match the female sexual capacity. He also fears the alteration of consciousness that can come through orgasm or may be unable to experience it. She must then avoid an aftermath in which she is open to all persuasion; immature males see their opportunity to manipulate mentally when the woman is defenceless. Another factor is that the woman has powerful sexual highs during the course of her cycle, and unless she has got them organized with the help of the menstrual mandala they may take her unawares. The male will find using the mandala that his best sexual capacities coincide with those of his woman partner.

So the first rule is to find the contours of one's sexual energy with the menstrual mandala. Most women have a particular high at ovulation (very definitely not the 'safe' time) and a possibly greater high at menstruation. There is often a very intense auxiliary high at pre-menstrual. Each quadrant of the cycle has its own particular sexual quality; there may be a subsidiary high at the beginning of the cycle, almost like the energy of a fresh beginning.

A second rule is that there is nothing better than sex for crossing transition thresholds with energy, consciousness and excitement. But this does mean *consciousness*; that is, an attention to the mental side of sex and its altered states, each of which will have a quality from its place in the cycle. Thus sex at ovulation with the likelihood of impregnation has an enfolding and nesting feeling. Pre-menstrual sex is like dealing with a trembler switch on a booby-trapped body: you must both proceed with knowledge and extreme delicacy if the energy of that exploding bomb which is the unfertilized egg (or the regressing corpus luteum) is to be harnessed and shared by both.

Sex at ovulation, if it is not intended to impregnate, puts energy into the cycle, and with its total body-feeling reduces the separation-anxiety of travelling into the separation phase. The energy of sex at the pre-menstrual time dissolves anticipatory transition depression of the period, precisely because its preceding pre-menstrual stage has been *enjoyed* so thoroughly.

Equally, sex at menstruation, full of strange archaic images and atavistic feelings, can people that time with multitudes of creative ideas and images which, with the trust that they will come again next month, can be bid adieu as one moves to the next state of a new cycle's beginning. Some of those treasures carry their energy right through the ovulation and subsequent stages, and this is the beginning of full unity of the cycle.

The man's inner self will be following these changes whether he likes it or not, and he can choose whether or not to open himself to them. The testosterone-provoked brain-lateralization model says that excitement itself will stimulate the secretion of more testosterone, making the immature male even more left-brained, but impelling him towards sex which, if he is capable, can give him an opportunity to enter the right-brain state. This is his great transition. However, responding to testosterone arousal creates more testosterone which then inclines him to become macho and left-brained again. He can break out of that oscillation only by guiding his hormones by means of changing attitudes.

The new attitudes will be less macho, regarding the woman as more of a leader in sexuality (this is not the same as domination; the bedroom is no place for competitive attitudes). He must also understand the way women have been put down in history, and how they are far different from the conventional images purveyed by male culture. He is not to fear this, but to be responsive to the sheer beauty of spontaneous feminine imagery in dreams and fantasies, and to their power. Creativity between partners always combines listening with telling. Sex can be a form of not listening too. The man who prides himself on being able to continue lovemaking for a couple of hours, giving the woman repeated orgasms until she can take no more, and finally ejaculating into her unresponsive openness, is killing some dragon of his own, probably a maternal menstrual one. A physical sexual capacity of this order should be the norm for most men who are reasonably fit, but the attitude of a lover of women will be worlds apart from it. Real lovers watch out for the individual character of each love-making.

At multi-orgasmic time, say menstruation, lovers can carefully nurture response so that an orgasm appears by manipulation of the clitoris at the end of foreplay, then another orgasm or peak perhaps with shallow penetration; the man must retain here during the woman's plateau, and then gently stimulate her to a new peak, while he retains; then perhaps his excitation will fall, which she must stimulate to the point where he can give her another peak, during which he peaks too, but without ejaculating. A traditional pattern given in the eastern love-books is perhaps four peaks (not counting clitoral peak) to the point where the partners' mutual desire is overwhelming, and they have a terminal climax together. Ancient texts say that the woman is best on top during menstruation, and then she is a 'doorway to the other worlds'.

During this entire time there will have been a continual interplay of sensations with feelings with mental images in a kind of streaming. Though this is always individual to particular lovers and can only be described in the greatest poetry, what goes on parallel to and increasing with the various 'peaks' or 'climaxes' could properly be called the 'orgasm'. It gathers during the love-making and does not disappear after a climax, but persists as the 'afterglow', often during the next day and beyond. It is a wonderful feeling of well-being, combined with sharpness of perception and deepness of thought-feeling. The orgasm eroticizes the world for both partners. It is timeless, egoless, and in continuum with nature. It is a kind of lightening or enlightenment of the body. This of course is the great experience – none of us can expect it to happen every time. But once having experienced it, like an enlightenment in Zen or a conversion in a religion, there is a permanent change.

Men feel handicapped because after their ejaculation there is a refractory period when they often can't bear to be touched. It is necessary to separate the climax from the ejaculation, and the ability to do this is one of the great benefits of Hatha and Taoist yoga. If men can do this – that is, delay the ejaculation – they will find they experience a number of mini-climaxes in response to the climaxes of the woman. This is the 'staircase' described above. At the end, after many inner events on both sides, there is a point of no return for both partners, and a final mutual climax together. Both will then probably have a refractory period (the woman's due to a deep 'womb-climax') and neither will require any further stimulation though touch, cuddling, will have a changed quality and will merge with sleep and dreams.

Many people have these experiences, but for others they may seem a counsel of perfection. We can only say this is the kind of thing that happens as the partners become familiar with the menstrual rhythm. It is important to remember that there is always a time during the cycle when the woman is not interested in sex; she should not be persuaded into intercourse by a partner or a set of circumstances. This point can move round the cycle, but it frequently positions itself in the late luteal phase, as we said above, say around Day 21, just at the time of the 'death of the egg' and early premenstrual sniffles.

Sex is the most advanced form of yoga available to most people; it is, as it were, one's taste of 'The Domain of Heaven and Earth'. As in yoga, relaxation is of prime importance. If a couple can reach the conjoined orgasm described above, they are likely to be carried away into sleep and dreams, and will only remember the waking up, which can be like being reborn. Barriers will have gone down; the boundaries of the body will seem to have been dissolved. It is the deepest meditative state most people can achieve. As with any other contact with the unconscious, it is possible to make requests and ask questions in such a state of reverie, or whole-brain state (remember, there is evidence that brain lateralization shifts in the man after orgasm). It is like a prayer. Speak into the mystery, and the mystery answers. Questions or requests made in this trance-state will receive answers, either by a show of imagery, or by a thought coming into one's mind much later. We have known painters who in this state can watch their paintings in progress change to a more advanced stage. Either or both partners can make a request in this manner, with or without the knowledge of the other. The relaxation is wonderful to explore for its own sake, supposing one has not plunged into post-coital sleep. One's attention explores the body from head to toe from *inside*, finding it full of ample rooms and unanticipated beauties. A simple non-sexual imaging to remember this feeling is to explore every bone of one's skeleton, imagining that each bone is turning to shining gold.

Undoubtedly a woman has a more direct and natural connection to these experiences than a man has. One of the most popular of current sex books in America speaks of the cultivation of 'psychasms'[4] – the word is coined on the analogy of 'orgasm' being of the organism, 'psychasm' of the mind. The man is directed in a languorous and meditative way towards acts that will excite him, but not too rapidly and explosively. Stroking the frenulum (the little furrow that interrupts the penile glans) and the raphe (the apparent joint of the two halves of the scrotum) is recommended. This is fine as far as it goes, but in our opinion the first rule for the man is to recognize the woman's strong menstrual sexual rhythm, and ride on that. His own rhythms will then begin to develop, and give feedback to the woman's. Without this, the sexual cycle will be disjointed.

The man should take exercise, but it should not be competitive exercise which leads to macho patterns of sexuality. The soldier, as it were, after killing in battle, 'wipes his sword', that is, has sex. Or he may be trained by the ethos of competitive sports to a phallic insensitivity – 'giving the woman her orgasm' until he finally and triumphantly ejaculates into her, not with her. Yoga and T'ai Chi (remembering, however, that the latter was in origin a martial art) are fine. Exercise which experiences and does not clench the man into blind effort is needed. Walking is one of the best forms of exercise – and one most often walks *with* other people rather than against them.

With regard to separating climax and ejaculation, he can, with yoga, learn the *bandhas*, which are contractions of the musculature of the throat and of the pelvic diaphragm which are said to seal the energy within the body. Since 'energy' equals 'awareness' in yoga, the *bandhas* make one more aware of normally unconscious events in the sealed areas, and increase control. The *Asvini mudra* and *mula bandha* are contractions of the anus and then of the whole lower pelvic diaphragm which make a man more aware of his approaching ejaculation, so he can push back the 'point of no return'. In Canadian work on teaching men for multi-orgasms, devices like the ECG have been used for this kind of training; also the woman may feel it coming before the man does, and can warn him!

These *bandhas* – providing there is no medical reason for not learning them – need to be taught in a class with an experienced teacher or from a good yoga book. The *jalandhara bandha* of the neck-muscles has the effect of stimulating the gentling parasympathetic nervous system through the carotid plexus. This gentling allows the man to attend better to events in his body; also, like the other *bandhas*, it helps to control ejaculation. It also 'raises energy', that is, it stimulates erogenous zones which are often neglected: the throat, the nipples and the whole ribcage. Many men ejaculate simply from the penis, while it is common for a woman to climax from a touch on any part of the body. These exercises help give a man that womanly sensitivity; and, as we say, the ability to have, like the woman, several climaxes without ejaculation, while the orgasm assembles and amplifies its energies beyond and behind the climaxes.

The two constitutions – male and female – are not too dissimilar after all. The woman can have a succession of climaxes, each of which carries strong and increasing orgasmic feeling. She may have a partner who can bring her on to her terminative climax, which will release her into the orgasmic state, which is sensitive, vulnerable and visionary; though it may be full of extroverted energy, especially if she is drawing upon pre-menstrual energy. Her terminative climax may coincide with her partner's seminal emission that may either be ejaculatory within her or, as it were, drawn from him like milking. There are indications that the woman may also emit urethral fluid. In the man, the ejaculation is usually terminative and hopefully orgasmic as the last climax in the series, though younger men may have enough fluid to start up the sequence again more than once; and the woman can discover behind the climax she thought terminative further climaxes.

On the way, a man may have several climaxes without emission, which are increasingly orgasmic; or his climaxes may be felt in the whole body as if drawn up from the penis. This matches the female pattern: successive climaxes appear to rise in the body, from the clitoris to the vagina and womb with deeper penetration, and seemingly higher to involve the whole body in an altered state of feeling. It is this 'altered state' of feeling and consciousness, with its visionary experience and streaming sensations as though a person were immersed in life's flow, for which we reserve the term 'orgasmic'. 'Climax' is a peak sensation usually accompanied by involuntary muscular contraction whose further dimension is orgasmic. It may be succeeded by orgasmic feeling even if congress is not continued to the partners' ultimate conclusion, hence the occasional success of 'quickies'. The climaxes generate or discover the orgasm. Orgasmic feeling is 'erotic' feeling, as opposed to sexual sensation, and the purpose of sex without reproduction is to transform sexual sensation into erotic living. Erotic living is like the most passionate creative feeling coupled with a profound relaxation and openness. Perhaps it is our natural state. It can be opened to us in a lesser degree by hypnosis, relaxation or meditation. It can be achieved without sexuality at all; though in hypnosis a caress and a suggestion, or some involvement of the non-visual sense is mandatory. 'Mesmerism' is like the state of being in love; a wholebrain, whole-body state, in which whatever one requires from oneself can be forthcoming. The achieved menstrual state is like that, as is the state of being serenely pregnant. Subject and object at once.

It was the original position of Anton Mesmer[5] that his method was in truth the establishing of a continuum with the whole environment, including weather, tides and planets. In the nineteenth century the mesmeric state was often entered voluntarily and for many months at a time, and there are contemporary accounts of people becoming their best selves by this means. Such states of consciousness are a continuum stretching from the heights of insight, vision, creativity and productive living, to the depths of corruption. It depends what we want to make of it. Many call it happiness, but our politics is too corrupt for that word. It is 'afterglow', but the word is too cosy. 'Trance' is suspect. It is so familiar yet so tabooed that in English there is no word for it.

It is also as though the orgasmic/erotic state moves towards us as we move towards it, like the other invocations and evocations of the 'unconscious' we have suggested in this book. It is as though we have kept the body unconscious as well as the mind. Or as if that erotic energy was latent in various places in the body, and the body protested under the pressure of possibilities unfulfilled. So we called it PMS and the like, for it is women who are initially most gifted in these things. What God or demon separated religion and sexuality, the highest aspiration of people from their greatest sympathetic capabilities?

Trying to find words to serve the 'erotic' or 'orgasmic' points to how our sensibilities have become so corrupted that we have no language to describe and communicate these experiences. Scientific language is off-putting and misdirecting, as has been scientific research on these matters. Poetry is regarded as mere metaphor, instead of an exact feeling-description. Thus are feeling and thought separated, even though they are natural companions, especially in the sexual act. A symbolic description will actually tune the feelings from both sides, as the erotic and the mundane consensus draw together. Advice to men as how best to achieve the generation of 'bliss-waves' is neatly summarized in a Tibetan text.[6] The man should cultivate the Four Techniques; which are Downward Motion; Retention; Backward Motion; and Saturation. Downward motion 'is like a smith hammering a metal mirror, making the four types of delight descend slowly, like a tortoise, from the head to the sexual region, so realising the delights in their natural order'. Retention 'is to hold the delight as one would a lamp in a storm'. Backward motion 'is like an elephant drinking water, making the four joyous delights ascend to the head region and keeping them stable'. Saturation 'is like a farmer watering his crops, very carefully to ensure that every pore of the skin is saturated with the consummation of love'.

The Hindu Tantric system of sexual religion has its own menstrual mandala – organized with exact descriptions of the spreading and contraction of the erogenous zones through the menstrual cycle. We in the West have had until now nothing comparable, as we have neglected and tabooed the cycle for so long. It is strange and gracious that this being – let us say, as with symbols 'this goddess' – is still willing to come forward. It is no use adopting another culture's symbology wholesale. The West has to make its own foundation studies in some simple basic menstrual mandala, such as the one we have offered. We have to use the symbology that is offered to us in these early negotiations by the other side itself, the so-called unconscious, in our dreams and waking dreams and creative explorations. Then we must return them over the net, as it were, to our facing partner, and see by her response whether we have understood the message properly, returned the stroke effectively. As we say – 'Symball Tennis'.

Men are sometimes stuck with a symbology that is inconvenient and which is also called, rather unsympathetically, a paraphilia or fetish. Paraphilias must be submitted to the relationship. Women, in their changing flow, are less prone to these things. Most people have a trace of them, called sympathetically, and returning the stroke correctly, a 'turn-on'. Male turn-ons can be compulsive, and great sympathy is needed from the female partner if whatever-it-is happens not to be a turn-on for her. It is quite likely, however, that at some time in the cycle it can turn her on as well.

There is a range here from a preference for certain garments (which everybody has an opinion about and is the way one develops and responds to a style of dress), through a complex and powerful turn-on, like wearing elaborate underwear for sex. It may be a further turn-on to wear it in public under an ordinary dress. This is a kind of foreplay in which it is difficult to accuse anybody of 'fetishism'. The man will be turned on by the garments, in bedroom or street, and this will turn on the woman, who will see the erotic point from that moment if she hasn't seen it before. This will further turn on the man, in that delightful staircase or wave of bliss or positive feed-back situation.

At the other end of the spectrum is the rather sad and delicate situation when the lover is incapable of sexual excitement without the 'fetish', commonly articles of adornment, clothes, footwear, feet or hair. The part stands for the whole, and the whole is not visibly present. But here the fetish is a symbol like the other symbols involved in our lives. It is a magic, for the erotic spirit gains access through the symbolic object. It is probable that the symbol is derived in childhood from an inadvertent seductiveness during the menstrual cycle of the mother. Menstruation to the child can be so strong and contradictory – being both feared and desired – that the male child may actually become dissolved in his mother's near-birth atmosphere, so absorbing are the sensations and feelings that a powerfully menstruating woman emits. The fetish may be a kind of lover's keepsake of these times; such a profound experience that the psyche needs to keep a token of it which is also a door for re-entry.

So the paraphilia may be a way of tuning back into cycle-events. It probably developed as a symbolic expedient for passing thresholds in the difficult pre-menstrual atmosphere of a disturbed childhood home.

Working with the menstrual cycle along the lines we have suggested will bring consciousness to these areas, and may result in a great flowering-out of the symbol. So-called abnormal sexual practices correctly handled may yield up great power, and may appear, disappear and reappear altered, as psycho-sexual development continues. If a fetish or other paraphilia is a symbol of the man's childhood experience of menstruation, then the reason why women do not have them so often is that the woman has the cycle instead. In fact the fetish may be the thing that the passionate man holds on to, to make him independent of the changes in the woman. When he finds the eros that the cycle-changes can yield, then the fetish may dissolve and yield up its riches, or it may persist as a sexual variation and shed its symbolic light on loving encounters, giving them a strange and surreal emphasis. Extraordinary powers of eroticism in the man may be packed in the image. A man's intransigence against the period is a hanging-on in the face of change, so a fetishist is one better than a man who makes a fetish of masculinity. A fetish may be a man's chief right-brain thing. His practice may give him sexual strength; if it is masturbatory, his masturbation may sensitize him to his lover.

Sealed Writing

There is one other useful practice we'd like to discuss here: sealed writing. You simply write down whatever comes into your head for twenty minutes or so before you go to bed, or at another convenient relaxed time. You persist, whatever you think you have or have not written, or even if you find you can write no more than a single word again and again. Most important of all, you *do not read it* – yet. You persist for three months, or a full month at least. At the end of this time, you read it; better still, hand it to a trusted friend to read to you.

By this method you discover that there is something in you that speaks better than you know. In such a script there is always confusion, then, at its height, a relaxation, followed by a synaesthesia: the senses come together in the words and some beautiful image appears. Moreover, that image and its theme are likely to surface again and again, forming at last a coherent statement. Writers can lift out this new and precious system and allow it to develop by their normal working-methods. In any event, it is an important personal discovery. Language, which can handle all the senses, thought and feeling too, clears like a magic mirror to the supersensible, which includes one's inner senses and further personality. We have supervised hundreds of these scripts, and they have never failed to stimulate development in people who persist with the method. One must simply go at it with a 'willing suspension of disbelief'. It is linguistic yoga, using both the right- and left-brain modes of language.

It is a good idea, if you become stuck during the twenty minutes, deliberately to move the senses away from the eyes. As James Hillman says: 'The place of one's sensitivity may move from eye to ear and then through the senses of touch, taste, and scent, so that we begin to perceive more and more in particulars, less and less in overviews.'[7]

After a bit of practice, one can approach the exercise magically: that is, with an intention which may be put humbly to one's inner self as a request. One would say, 'Please allow me to know more of the secrets of my period,' and continue with the sealed writing. One's 'sealed writing' is the companion to all other right-brain exercises, in the sense that it will begin to pick up from everything one does.

17. Homoeopathy, Hypnosis, Acupuncture and Massage

Homoeopathy

Homoeopathy is not fringe medicine. It is a properly authenticated system of medical practice and observation administered by qualified physicians skilled in diagnosis who have gone further in their art and science than the manipulative and invasive medicine taught in medical schools. There is a very considerable body of knowledge which authenticates its effects, and a good theoretical basis for its cures. The record of its cures can match favourably that of 'scientific' medicine, and has done so for nearly three hundred years. It is different from herbalism, though it draws upon its wisdom and knowledge of woman-matters. It takes account of the mind and the emotions as well as of the body, and a homoeopathic examination, which may take an hour or more on the initial consultation, inquires into every aspect of the patient's life in order to build up a whole picture, which then has its remedy or series of remedies. If the diagnosis is correct, the effect can be miraculous and long-lasting. The remedies come from a very large repertory of substances which are given in high dilution, and the effect is more like an immune response than chemical intervention.

Homoeopathy is almost the first line of attack for PMS or POS, together with proper nutrition, dream-study and the use of the menstrual mandala or diary. But we urge the reader to consult only medically qualified homoeopaths who are properly registered with a reputable homoeopathic organization of long standing. There are many talented lay homoeopaths but we believe that it is better to consult a doctor who has *seen beyond* current medical practice from a close experience with it. Nor should one self-prescribe. Many stores now carry homoeopathic remedies, but indiscriminate use of these without the supervision of your homoeopath can erode the very sensitive response to your 'type remedy'. Allopathic doctors often see the homoeopathic doctor as an enemy; but, as in all woman's matters, one must ask the old question 'Who profits?' Homoeopathy, which uses naturally-occurring substances (not patented) that have no side-effects, if adopted by the medical profession, as it should be, would put sectors of the drug firms and the hospitals out of business. Beware the doctor who is not a committed homoeopath, but who has simply taken a certificate as a sop to his more enlightened patients, and actually prefers to use synthetic medicines and surgery to effect his cures.

One is likely to find that the taking of the remedy – usually a small white pill – and the whole interesting ceremony of consulting the homoeopath, starts up a dream-sequence. Dreaming and the immune system prove to be intimately connected; there will be a homoeopathic or immune response which may be an 'aggravation' – that is, a short-lived intensification of the trouble – which is an excellent sign, and probably a strong reverie or dream to go with it. The dream, if menstrual distress is being treated, will undoubtedly have a menstrual content, which consulting the menstrual mandala will help illuminate. But it must be remembered that what happens menstrually happens to the whole constitution; the menstrual response is a kind of diagnostic window.

There is one homoeopathic remedy that your doctor will probably allow you to use in the home quite freely, and that is the Bach Rescue Remedy. This was specially designed for shock following an injury, but it will also reduce dream-shock if you are expecting bad dreams pre-menstrually; or after a bad dream that is difficult to remember, three drops of the remedy in a few ounces of water, to be held in the mouth before swallowing, is effective (the mouth and particularly the root of the tongue are important sites of absorption). Remember that in dreaming, as in negotiating the cycle, the aim is to move easily from waking to rest and into the dream and out again with as much recall as possible.

Hypnosis

Again, in the hands of a properly qualified and experienced practitioner, and if it suits you, the waking-dreaming state of hypnosis can have almost miraculous results – from resetting an irregular cycle towards a more comfortable rhythmical mode, to opening up the conscious mind to dreams and to interesting feeling-change perceptions in the body. This is an area to which our remarks about trance and reverie also apply, especially if you can ease your passage across thresholds and into and out of these altered states by asking your hypnotist to give you training for self-help or auto-hypnosis.

The hypnotic state is an exceedingly pleasant one, like the way one can float between waking and dreaming, and in it the conscious and unconscious minds can learn to catch up with each other, as it were, and co-operate. In this state one is in an enhanced condition, not a diminished one, and it is a condition of extraordinary sensitivity. This is why one must seek an experienced practitioner who has trained properly, and who knows how to put the benefits of hypnosis squarely in the hands of her/his client for their own use.

Acupuncture, Massage and its Forms

As we have said, there is a lot of knowledge of women's matters neglected by 'medical science', or reserved in certain other areas. Acupuncture, like homoeopathy, treats the individual as a whole and can result in an almost miraculous relief of PMS, POS and menstrual cramps. Acupuncture is well worth a try. Find a properly qualified acupuncturist, one who offers treatment with new, unused needles. A session is likely to produce vivid dreams and fantasies.

Menstrual distress can be seen in acupuncture treatment as a concentration or stagnation of energy in one area. It is as though the needles, inserted at the appropriate acupuncture points, are like taps which cause this energy to flow through channels called 'meridians'. This is like the free flow of energy which unifies the cycle itself.

There are small 'no needles' home acupuncture kits now on sale which work on batteries. These can be effective and are well worth a try.

Shiatsu is a form of Japanese massage that uses pressure on points along these same meridians. The idea is to *balance* these forces, as in acupuncture. Again, there can be a miraculous-seeming effect. The experience of touch in the massage, and the stimulation of the non-visual senses is also likely to result in dreams and vivid waking imagery, and these of course should be noted.

Reflexology is a related therapy which is a massage of the points and channels of the hands and feet. It can be learnt and practised at home. Reflexology can be inexpressibly consoling and comforting if it is performed by a willing partner just *before* any menstrual trouble is expected, as charted by the mandala. It is sometimes very easy to find the points that are tender just as the swelling of PMS or POS begins. Massaging this tenderness gives the energy that helps move the cycle past this threshold. Tenderness and atmosphere is created and love-making, the best of all massages, may naturally follow. In foot reflexology there is a point at the back of the ankle in the Achilles tendon that may sometimes bring the period on, particularly if combined with a correct leg-massage.

Reflexology and Shiatsu treatment are now on the therapy lists of most alternative health centres, and so it is quite easy and inexpensive to get advice and tuition, which then can be used at home.

There are various systems of massage, but we recommend the Do-In pattern.[1] Again, there are excellent books, and the practice can be very detailed, or can be simplified and used as a pattern of caress with pauses at tender places. The pattern is a kind of spiral starting with the hands and ending with the navel, and creates a movement of energy that helps all bodily functions.

The hands are treated first, kneading along the bones and lines, then the wrists, then down the inside and up the outside of the arm, paying attention to the funny-bone point an inch or so below the elbow, and the one on the bone on the outside surface under the biceps. Then the head and the face are massaged in ways which feel agreeable, including the ears. The nape of the neck follows, and the shoulders, the chest is tapped all over, up the breastbone and down the outside of the ribs, and massaging between the ribs (which will feel ticklish). Then there is a pause to let the breathing settle in its new pattern, because finding a new, fuller, easier breath is part of massage. Breath is responsive to all things conscious and unconscious just as the cycle itself is. Good rhythm with the one often means good rhythm with the other.

After this the feet are massaged, with particular attention paid to a relaxing and energizing point at the inside root of the big toes; then the ankles, with particular attention paid to any tenderness in the Achilles tendon. The legs are massaged down the outside, up the inside (these directions of flow on the upper and lower limbs are most important) and one should seek to massage *inside* the edges of the tibia (there is an energizing point one can find on this edge four fingers below the knee-socket), massaging downwards; and within the edges of the tibia as one returns upwards, pressing as well into the fleshy calf-muscles. The thighs need kneading, and behind the knees; the bones of the pelvis need to be felt out agreeably, and the iliac crest massaged, the kidneys and back rubbed upwards, and then the front down to the navel. This needs to be rubbed spirally, both ways. This is a simple pattern which, done gently in turn, will give much pleasure and relief. The book cited will fill out the above description.

One should massage to give pleasure, and to relax, and one should not probe hard anywhere there is a pain, or where there is a wart or a mole. If there is tenderness on legs, arms, hands or feet, it must be massaged only as if it can be massaged away. Continue only if the slight pain shifts into pleasure.

Some partners may find themselves sensitive enough to the flow of body-currents to use forms of polarity massage, which is simply balancing and equalizing energies in the body by providing channels through another body. Thus a hand on the forehead and at the nape of the neck will often remove a headache. Many people find that a current seems to flow. People who are fortunate enough to be able to perceive these currents from body to body will want to practise to feel them during sex, which is the equilibrating massage *par excellence*.

The skin is the second biggest organ of the body – the first is the liver – and it is the organ of that sense we have made so unconscious, touch. Without touch, we cannot be in touch – especially with the menstrual cycle. The skin is electrical as the brain. Attach an EEG machine to the scalp and you can see brain-waves; but you can also attach electrodes to the skin and see the pulsations of conductance and resistance that play through it with every emotion; it is a great organ of the unconscious mind. Of course one must balance these currents through it, and before one becomes too sensitive in the cycle too. After a massage that has got the currents right, you feel as though your skin can see from inside. This can happen naturally in sex, in the 'skin orgasm', but if it doesn't come naturally, then massage will help. The whole-body massage can of course be done with the correctly chosen oil. If one's partner is male, this oil, say for PMS, will be as right for him as it is for you.

18. Relaxation Practice Outline

1. Lie comfortably, but not as for ordinary sleep. This is a special state, between sleeping and waking. Usually we plunge straight into sleep, and wake up suddenly too, so we know little of the events that occur during the transition. This transition between sleeping and waking, between conscious processes and unconscious wisdom, is the creative state. One can lie on the floor, the neck slightly propped, the body covered with a blanket. The skin becomes very relaxed, silky and warm, so one must conserve heat.

2. Select a spot or crack on the ceiling, a little above one's eyes' normal level of sight. Stare at this spot, without blinking. Let it be the only visible thing in the world, and let your attention flow between you and the spot. But *at the same time* remind your body what it feels like to go to sleep, the limbs heavy and warm, the sinking and floating feeling, and how the eyes, when one is sleepy, insist on closing. Allow your open eyes to feel this wish for sleepy closing, but do not allow them to close yet.

3. Continue to remind your body of how it feels to sleep peacefully and let the sleepy feeling increase in your eyes until they cannot remain open, and drop of their own accord. As they close, feel the small pleasant shock of transition between waking world of light and the warm sleepy darkness in your own head and body.

4. Now, with the eyes always closed, attend to your big toe on the left foot. Don't move it, just know it is there. Feel its existence, the space it occupies, its warmth. Now do the same for your right big toe. Allow this gently focused awareness to spread to your other toes, and then to the soles of your feet, the heels, and slowly to the whole foot. You can now feel the touch of the whole skin of your foot. Be aware of the warmth of it too, and the heaviness.

5. Allow the feelings of warmth, heaviness and touch to spread inward, so that you seem to feel the bones relaxing, melting to the

touch. Let the warmth and relaxation spread up to the ankles, the shins, the calves of the legs, slowly, warmly and gently, to the knees and to the thighs with their weight, and the buttocks that feel the warm weight of the floor pressing upwards. Let the flood of warmth and relaxation and awareness spread over your belly and over the small of your back. Let the bones of your pelvis melt, and let the warmth and the relaxation travel up your back and over your shoulder-blades like warm soft dark hands caressing. Let it travel over your chest, where the breath is coming and going of its own accord, without you having to do anything to help it. Let the relaxation travel to your neck, and soften your jaw-line, and to the back of your neck, and soften it there. Let it travel down your left arm, warming it in sections, melting the bones, and travel out of your fingers, which are so relaxed they seem to stretch far out into the distance. And from the right shoulder down the right arm and out of the fingers. Let it travel over your face, which simply rests without expression on its bones, serene as the face of a buddha. Allow the space between the eyebrows to widen, and the brow to become broader, and be soothed by soft warm hands, and the relaxation to travel over the scalp like warm oil spreading under the hair. If there are thoughts or pictures flashing now, let them come, and then let them go, and allow the relaxation to spread over the back of the head down the nape of the neck and down the spine, as though there were a tap at the base of the spine, and it was open, and all tension was draining away to the centre of the earth.

6. Now attend only to the breathing. Watch it come and go slowly of its own accord, as it will. Breath is the link between conscious and unconscious, the door; for we can consciously direct our breath or, as now, allow it to come and go as it will. Breath responds to the whole universe inside you, and outside you. Knowing your breathing, you are both subject and object.

7. Only pay more attention to the out-breath, which is the relaxing breath. Feel your relaxation deepen a little more each time you breath out. Now imagine that you are breathing out an inch or two below your navel. Let the breath come out at this place, which seems open. You may feel a warmth there as you do this, or a tingling. Allow any thoughts or dream pictures to come, look at them, let them go, and return to your breath, your breath that is coming and going of its own accord, an inch or so below your navel, and relaxing you further with each out-breath. Stay in this very pleasant place as long as you have determined.

8. When you are ready, imagine you are a diver, ready to return by your own buoyancy from a great depth to the light above. Count backwards from twenty as you come up from those depths, pausing occasionally to remember them, and think that your eyes will open as you reach the number 'one'.

9. Open your eyes, and move very gently, carefully at first. Think about what has happened. Take notes very gently, for things alter as you move.

Many people have remarkable experiences involving imagery, waking dreams, sudden vivid insights, and the sheer unexpected pleasure of deep relaxation the first time they try this method. Generally speaking, it is best to promise oneself to do it every day for about twenty minutes or more for a fortnight. That gives it a chance. We have shared this technique with some hundreds of people, and everybody who has given it this chance reports considerable benefits: in dream-recall, creativity, improved health, and alleviation of menstrual distress. Everybody alters the sequence and the details to suit themselves as they become practised. Often one can start with an intention, such as a puzzling dream and a request for illumination, forget the intention while initiating the relaxation, and recall it again while doing the 'womb-breathing' (men included). Often then the re-dreaming or solution is seen as in a magic mirror of the out-breath in the lower abdomen.

You can make a tape-recording to listen to while relaxing, and re-record as you find the instructions that suit you best.

Remember at the beginning, if you are doing relaxation by yourself (or recall it to anybody you are guiding into relaxation), that it is very easy to wake up from this relaxation if there is any emergency. It is best, however, to take the phone off the hook. If somebody you are guiding wishes to remain 'down there' and resists returning, you can ask them why. They usually say 'It's so nice . . .' and one should let them stay there. It will sometimes develop into a brief nap. In any case, the relaxation is very refreshing. One should gently accustom oneself to taking simple notes, as part of the menstrual mandala.

Afterword:
Towards a Summary

Dreaming follows the four-fold structure of the cycle as measured by hormone levels: there are ovulation, pre-menstruation, menstruation and pre-ovulation dreams. Each stage has its characteristic images or symbols, which direct attention to the disposal of one's psychological and physical energy; participation in the dream increases knowledge of oneself and others.

These significant images are not exclusive to the stations of the cycle, but they are typical of that station. The images form patterns of relationship and transformation. The pre-menstrual and pre-ovulation thresholds require adjustment or transformation to pass consciously, and these are particularly sensitive according to one's current disposition towards ovulatory values or menstrual values, which appear to correspond broadly to right-brain and left-brain values. Passing them consciously tends to reduce menstrual distress, sometimes radically.

The aim is an overview of the cycle leading to wholeness and an ability to draw on its alternating energies, to possess it rather than to be possessed by it. This synthesis of the two opposites to a new spirit combining both may be the culmination of menopause. The cycle is then seen as a series of alchemical distillations resulting in illumination.

Men's dreams, and children's too, are responsive to the cycle. Men, who *may* have a three-month testosterone cycle of their own, though this is not certain, are more usually entrained by the strength of the woman's rhythm. However, they sometimes show an underlying cycle learnt in their families from their mothers and sisters. It is unfortunate when this 'shadow-cycle' contradicts, as it were, the manifest contemporary cycle of their living partner of the present day. Then it may happen that when that woman partner is ovulating, the man in contradiction or compensation, has menstrual emotions and desires; or when the partner is menstruating, then the man's shadow-cycle may declare ovulation interests, a desire for children, and sorrow that his partner is menstruating and is not pregnant. This conflict is the source of a lot of sorrow and difficulty in the home, and may be one of the basic causes of POS and PMS.

It is clear that such a collision of values in the home can result in much unhappiness, physical and mental; it was just such a collision of values that resulted in the taboo on this whole double-quadrant of woman's experience, since all the main world religions at the present time elect for ovulation-values. Woman is to be Mother, and that is all. The persistence of this view naturally leads to darkness and conflict in women's dreams and it is personal work on these that can lead out of menstrual unhappiness, since every mental discovery is accompanied by a physical change.

If your psyche is in conflict whether from inner or outer causes, then that exquisitely sensitive menstrual rhythm will be affected. If you find your way through as the dreams indicate, then a new clarity will come to the menstrual rhythm. Among the important archetypal figures is the pagan or witch, which represents woman's unacknowledged 'magical' powers, her 'human weather' and her connections with nature, which are seen as threatening and dangerous. It is a very common and frightening dream, often at ovulation separation time, that one is arrested, tried and burnt as a witch. This is ovulation's view of menstruation: it is witchy. There are frequent conflicts between old witch and young witch. This points to a basic family conflict to which great attention should be paid, between mother and daughter. As the young daughter reaches her puberty and begins to establish her rhythm, she thereby challenges the established rhythm of the living house, the source of which has been the mother. All kinds of subtle glandular and other field effects must be involved here. It is at the daughter's puberty that a mother begins to feel strongly that she is growing older, and indeed, the child's powerful glandular influences, perhaps mediated by pheromones, may entrain the maturation process in adults, so that they begin to grow into the next life-stage of middle-age. There will be dreams confirming this too.

The two main powers in the cycle are ovulation and menstruation, which begin by opposing each other. The difficulties mainly occur – expressed by PMS and POS – in entering or leaving these two states. Good nutrition and dreaming can help ease this passage.

Just as the changing hormones can influence the dreams, so the dreams can influence the hormones, and a knowledge of the typical dream-images and adventures can alter the physical pattern of the cycle. Thus willingly entering the dream-country armed with a knowledge of its inhabitants is to accept and be aware of that country and its customs; it is to accept oneself. As in visiting any other country with which one is not perfectly familiar, one is in a learning process and one is not there to swagger or show off, but to accept advice in a reasonable spirit.

Thus, if one has a dream of a schoolroom, and one is a teacher, one should resist feeling responsible for taking the class. The proper attitude is to sit quietly in one of the desks and wait for the teacher to arrive.

If one is offered sexual intercourse with a dream figure, one should not trouble oneself with feelings of loyalty to one's sexual partner in the outer world. He or she is not concerned with this; the dream figure who invites you to love is yourself, and this is a figure of the closest personal integration – perhaps this dream will result in the closer co-operation of the two sides of the cycle, two sides of the brain, the masculine and feminine within.

Dreaming is a sexual act in that during it the dreamer is excited.[1] The dream is a kind of afterglow to this inner conjunction. It is a whole-brain function, or can be, in which body and mind are united in creative, spontaneous and meaningful imagery. We must let Frank Avray Wilson have the last word on this state of afterglow or 'mesmerism' and how it relates to good living. He says one can train one's dreaming

> to the point where an incipient dreaming occurs in the midst of living, and all things become subtly transfigured by the light of dreams, which is the condition most primitives live in, and is the condition nature intended humans to enjoy incessantly ... The point is that the dream should not be interpreted in terms of ordinary reality, but rather, this reality in terms of the dream.

Concerning repression, he says: 'One does not become enlightened by imagining figures of light, but by making the darkness conscious.'[2]

Appendix: Various Dreamers' Experience of the Cycle

Please read the following with a sense of the actuality of dreams; and also the actuality of the bodily changes which are occurring in synchrony with the dreams. Try to relate the images with dreams of your own. In feeling into these images, or your own, relaxation to take you into a calm, picturing state is useful.

Each individual dream can be read as if it were a short vivid poem, like a Japanese haiku. The whole sequence could be read like the skeleton of an impressionistic short story. However you do it, the important thing is to take a creative and receptive attitude, and to bear in mind your own varying rhythms of the cycle. To do these things will lead to more dreams and further creativity.

Menstrual Domain Dreams

DAY 1
The man dreamed: 'All the electrical appliances were going of themselves.' In the morning his partner's period had come, and she had dreamed of a beautiful impossibility, a 'rainbow under the water'.

Another woman dreamed that she was caught in a crystal, but the dark face that was looking in on her was her rescuer, Lord Krishna, a very positive menstruous animus with the power to release her from the glass prison.

Another found a scant period after that night's dream of 'a game show, men in a line pulling ropes, one man very ugly, a lumpy nose, and ill-co-ordinated. The Master of Ceremonies says to me (him?), "You are doing well even though you are ill." The man looks ill and sad, but goes on with the game.'

A man on Day 1 had nightmares: 'The drains have backed up

with pieces of baby.' He dreamed again: 'The pipes high on the wall may be leaking. I can't make the coupling firmer until I screw opposite ways.'

DAY 2
The night of Day 2 gave this woman 'a complete narrative dream of delivery into the care of a powerful black menstrual man after many adventures of entering water and being able to breathe it, and setting underwater many explosions to destroy enemy structures.' The feeling of rebirth lasted through the day.

Another had dreams of difficult magic, an old Shaman's potion swirled in a cup, and reported that she had colonized her menstrual side by understanding its dreams, and now the former menstrual distress had moved to ovulation time. Among these wonderful menstrual dreams was 'a Candlemass celebrated blazing with candlelight, and the dark Lord Krishna came again and made love to all the women simultaneously – dark Lord of the Ladies.' Again it was the new moon.

Another woman found herself Mrs Superwoman at the period now instead of at ovulation; now the late cycle menstrual distress had gone, she dreamed of 'red mud, red dress, a touch felt and not seen that turned into love-making', her partner still not visible. Again it was the new moon.

DAY 3
This woman dreamed she was 'taught Gossip or Godspeech by dead Grandmother – this being a very helpful thing to have learnt.'

A man reports: 'She has her period – a sweet-smelling wet breath or vapour came from her. I had some nightmares. She had a restful night, but I am fighting with a bloody corpse – he is covered with blood – the upper part of the body which won't die.'

Another man dreamed on Day 3 that: 'A dead and living baby are present simultaneously – one waxes and the other wanes.'

Two women dream of passing new and different barriers: 'Blue plane, glider, testing cruise, we watch it fly over the field in sunlight. We go on our journey, guided by guides who are not as kind as they seem.' The other: 'A film studio, waiting at doorway eleven. Man collects me, takes me beyond a barrier prohibited to ordinary visitors.'

DAY 5
A man dreamed of milk boiling in a heavy iron saucepan with a cone in its centre to prevent it boiling over, looking like the pre-menstrual mandala. This was the day his partner's period stopped, a time of new beginnings. He thought his dream showed the cycle holding within itself the milk of ovulation being prepared, actively boiling.

DAY 6
This menstruator liked her period, and wanted to dwell there longer. She dreamed: 'A cave woman is showing me menstruation.'

Transition Dreams out of Menstruation

DAY 8
This woman reported as she moved out of her period: 'There were dreams now of the assessment of treasures and taking stock following after the great dreams of my previous pre-menstrual time. Now the treasures of the period were assembled ready to pass through to ovulation. The grip of the patriarchal ourobouros had untangled in a dream of finding a black garter snake on the veranda. This was the elemental energy separated from the incestuous situation.'

DAY 9
The fear of ovulation may shadow these days: 'I went from a place where I was with mother, relatives, to a shop where I wanted them to alter a skirt, shorten it, but the woman there is abusive, says she does not know me, suspects me of wrong-doing. Somewhere a child, a pram. Upset I leave the shop and go out, now it is dark, a dismal city, traffic, I cannot find my way home, I am lost, I cannot remember the name of the road I live in, I ask people but my crying upsets them and they go away.'

DAY 10
A woman who is mature but childless dreams an image of the entire cycle which comforts her as she enters her sterile ovulation: 'There is a gas fire, a sort of Rayburn. There is an image of a square in a circle. There is the elder sister of the mother, my loved aunt who

made a life without children and there is my mother and they are forging a wheel together on this Rayburn.'

A woman who might conceive prepares in her dream for ovulation: 'A girl or woman with fair hair, sitting down sketching a child-like drawing of a sailing ship which she has coloured in deep though not dark blue. She is very pregnant. Besides her stands her younger sister, a girl about twenty-three. This sister laughs and says, affectionately, "Aren't you silly?" The pregnant woman smiles.'

A man dreams of: 'A bloody hieroglyph, frightening, twice seen in different versions – then it was red life insurance certificate.'

DAY 11
In one dream a woman's calm transition to the green peace of ovulation is declared: 'Husband is doing counselling and is enjoying it in the College Library. I meet him on the headland path, he is happy with the work – I go to a big building to work, it is welcoming, I am quite happy. I ask the way in, a man tells me kindly up the steps – I work evenings. A man alone outdoors sitting on a grassy bank by a tree is looking over a valley – the path is blocked up leading round a hill. Then I see there is a way through on the near side but it has to be held up by wooden supports, it goes off to the right. I sit looking at the view, very green and sunlit, not taking the path yet (I have been along it before).'

Ovulation Domain Dreams

DAY 12
On Day 12 ovulation is about to begin, and she feels this is God's design. She sees a mandala of her cycle as if she was blessed: 'In a dark underground chamber with my husband, a sound like a huge iron trapdoor opening and then a feeling like a hand on my head and I know that this is God blessing us, that God came through the door; then I am very happy, and then God makes beautiful circular earrings in my ear lobes, a delicate cobweb design with pearl in centre.'

The transition to ovulation on Day 13 is seen by this woman's dream as a cross or crossing: 'A large cross or crucifix or big Christmas Tree which I put in the back of my car, a Station Wagon –

"Can you manage?" someone asks doubtfully. "Yes," I say confidently.'

DAY 13
And the male problem begins again for another woman as the ovulation-energies rise: 'A group of us are about to make a film, I am in a dingy bedroom, getting ready. A dark masculine young man, my chauffeur, wants me to go away with him and not make a film. He half begs, half bullies. He presses me down on the bed and lies on top of me, we have our clothes on, it is sexy. I don't know whether to go with him, or send him away.' Whatever her decision, the natural forces begin to burgeon: 'Later, in an overgrown garden, with many other people. Lifting up parts of a bush which has grown out over the pavements.'

DAY 14
Day 14, often the actual ovulation day, brings an image of the cycle as clothes cushioning a fall, of acceptance; the archetype shows the way: 'The great mother appearing with a black and white skirt and revolving and fluttering as she falls down the precipice of the cliff towards the sea. Her skirt buoys her up and she lands without harm, showing I can do it too.'

Another woman sees the whole cycle as an alchemical four-fold cooking process of 'squaring the circle' and her acceptance of it a synaesthesia in which a touch tastes: 'An old friend and I were together by an old square wooden box, actually a saucepan, it was bubbling and cooking, a thick dark blue saucepan, navy blue – the saucepan was square but I think it was round in the box. She put her hand in and tried to taste it with her hand and said, "I can taste it with my hand."'

Another woman dreamed on Day 14: 'It must have been my ovulation because I dreamed I was a big boat, and my daughter dreamed I was pregnant.'

This is a man's dream on Days 14 to 15 in a thirty-three-day cycle, when the hormone oestrogen would be peaking: 'A horse's activity followed the oestrogen curve. The horse's appearance altered with it too. A man and myself were going to draw this curve on the blackboard.'

DAY 15
This ovulation was on the full moon and brought a male dream-figure, a positive animus who was both famous singer and capable workman: 'Paul McCartney with some workmen, he up a ladder working. I say, early and on a Monday morning! Surprised to see him. Why not, he says. Over at the nearby university students stand on a balcony and mock the singer for posing as a workman. Should I go over there to explain? asks concerned singer.'

Post-Ovulation Dreams

DAY 15
This ovulation was an undesired and perilous event, the motherhood of the sea a dangerous one, monster-haunted: 'A huge field on which we, a group sparsely dispersed, are gathering harvest; weather clear but atmosphere of gloom. Field enormous, nothing else to be seen, it stretches to all horizons. I see a woman I recognize who is fat anyway, but now I see is pregnant. She is sulky, irritable, as we all are. Next, in procession, we (same group as in field?) are going along a high cliff path. In the sea, on our left, several ships (oil-rigs) are wrecked, men are desperately trying to climb on to the (orange-coloured?) steel of the wrecks; the sea is very turbulent, huge waves crashing. The men's cries for help reach us, we on the cliff are very upset; then a voice says, the sea snakes will get the men. Later, we complain about having to witness the shipwrecks; but are told (by an overseer, or intermediary) that we knew we were forbidden to watch along that section of cliffpath and should have worn blindfolds.'

DAY 16
Ovulation is passing, both regretted and desired – even the living child is dismissed – but the menstrual flowers make their imminent presence felt. 'On the lawn there are two giraffes – fighting. Their bodies are twisted and bound together, they are fighting to the death – my daughter is too close, she is kicked and falls to the ground – I'm by the winter flowerbed full of dead flowers and I see that the deep red geranium is beginning to flower and I am very pleased – I pick off the dead flowerheads and dead twigs to give the plant a good chance to flower more.'

Another woman enjoys the presence of the ideal husband and father, the ovulation animus: 'A concert, at first children, amateurs in costumes of animals, then a professional, a man, a singer, eminent. I see articles about him in Sunday papers. Afterwards I go with another man and speak to the singer. He says little, but has this strong presence. We say to him, down that way is an Indian restaurant, down there a Chinese. We go into the city, the buildings are beautiful, golden, calm.'

DAY 17
Ovulation is passing but a baby is dreamed – possibly the non-material child of menstruation: 'I was pregnant, about to have a baby. I felt one big contraction, cramping. I go down country lane, am driven to private hospital. The doctor talks to me, reminds me he delivered me of a child before. I say confidently, this time it will be different, easy.'

DAY 18
Ovulation is ending – there is no child – only the scar of the follicle on the ovary: 'Outside a school with a big round flowerbed cleared of plants. Well turned over brown earth, on one side the healed scar of a chopped-down tree. "Oh," I say sadly, "nothing is growing." The woman (headmistress?) says, "It will grow again."'

Pre-Menstrual Threshold Dreams

DAY 19
This woman's dream of post-ovulation was very explicit in its images: 'Had a dream of a corpus luteum seen as a green apple eaten.' She had also 'fallen off the roof' – that was falling off an ovulation high.

Another woman on the same cycle-day was still in her ovulation – the egg was still alive: 'Picking up a beautiful fat baby from his cot, white cot, he smiles, he is my son, he is too young to speak but he says, Mummy, Mummy, then some other words I can't remember. I'm at my parents' home, it's sunny everywhere, and I say to Dad, I never expected to have a second child, perhaps I'll even have a third. I laugh.'

A third woman started a streaming cold on this day – it seemed to her like suppressed weeping for the lost child.

DAY 20
Now ovulation begins to fear the oncoming menstrual state, its opposites and antagonists: 'In toilet, in semi-dark. Through window see a full congregation in church, singing. Fear they can see me. Fear their gloom and power. As if very old.'

DAY 21
The man shares the pre-menstrual threshold-passage: 'In a university – I am looking for a lavatory – there is a bedroom I have to go through for the lavatory. There is a guy whose room this is. I found the lavatory – there is a birthday cake stuck to the toilet seat, the underneath of the toilet seat – it's red and black with streaks of yellow.'

A woman sees the pre-menstrual energies in their animal form, and tames them in an image of her cycle: 'Cattle show. One shaggy long-nosed beast won't accept any young beast, won't mother them, drives them away. It says it hates them all. Says it is God. Then it is brought a young one. All at show are pleased. It comes from outer space and now we have it. I put some money carefully back into my bag. Then toys and toy animals on a revolving stand. I tidy them up.'

DAY 22
The menstrual standpoint is gaining hold as the dreamer separates from the ovulation domain – there is excrement but solidarity with women too; boundaries of convention are crossed: 'I went to a lesbian brothel. The brothel is a women's toilet, not very clean, women are going in and out using toilets – I inquire of a woman with dark hair and pale face. "It's £20," she says, "but no one's free to do it yet." "I haven't got £20, but I will get it and come back in the afternoon." My husband is away, I dance with women. I say "I haven't danced since my daughter was born." I say, "Yes, I am married, I like sex but I like this too." My husband comes in with a box of blue-and-white beautifully decorated stationery which he says is from the Holy Land. I am waiting, I think I understand why men go with prostitutes, it is so sexy.'

In another woman there is an eating-up of ovulation as she

makes her transition – the difficult action of putting ovulation behind one is eased with vivid imagery, and an unexpected delicious taste. She was at the funeral of a relative who did not exist; 'During the funeral the head of the corpse had been modelled by the caterers in sugar – very lifelike and the guests were given this to eat. The dead man's fingers were on the plate too and I took one of these and bit into it and it was delicious. There was a taste there.'

Dreams of teeth being removed or treated are frequent pre-menstrually, as though the tooth in the mouth symbolized the baby in the womb: 'Dentists, having my teeth filled, hardness of fillings in mouth, but sensation strongest of big complicated injection of opium or some other drug in my right arm. Resistance to drug then it overtakes me.'

DAY 23
One dreamer has a menstrual view of ovulation: 'Ann hands me a lettuce, icy from the freezer.'

DAY 24
Another dreamer sees the whole cycle in its four quadrants and accepts it as sustenance: 'She was frying vegetables – mostly mushrooms in a wok – but she'd divided the vegetables into two parts. She mixes all the vegetables together and then divides them into four parts very clearly, they mix as they fry.'

DAY 25
A woman dreams anticipating menstrual creativity: 'I am in a queue in a corridor, waiting. Lots of people wearing colourful, fine clothes to be presented in a grand room. Talking to a youngish man, a known poet. "Perhaps we are all artists, but we are not so important as the people in the next room." Talking, I say to the man and to the generality, "They say that we are artists so we must be rich and don't need money given to us." I say mockingly, "Of course I'm rich aren't you?" to the man. We laugh.'

DAY 26
This dreamer anticipates her period with a whole-cycle image of the red wine of menstruation and the white of ovulation: 'Geyser of red wine in bottle – clear white wine when poured.'

DAY 27

A woman sees in a dream how she may make her transition by a complete turn-around to an audience of helpful friends: 'There was a surface of a car park made with silver grey asphalt which actually moulded to her body – this was a moon colour.' She put her body and head right into it, was able to see from the back of her head two female friends comforting her.

This dreamer's period came without diarrhoea for the first time after this dream which distinguished excrement from menstrual blood: 'Then there was two yaks, one who was shit colour, the other one was menstrual colour. (Later on the shit had turned into chocolate.)' From the names of the animals maybe she still recoiled from both!

A man on this day dreamed: 'Wine! blood! killings by sword! zombies! house in decay! copper warriors!' and suffered a couvade with a feverish cold.

DAY 28

This was another man's couvade, dreamed of pre-menstrually by his wife: 'A grassy space between a wood and a lake, an extensive grassy space. My husband walks up to a stag who is with two or three deer – it is either spring or autumn and the deer are dangerous. He is diverting the animal energies which might otherwise attack me. He opens his coat like a flasher and the stag attacks him. They recede into the distance, there is a kind of roaring, but I don't know whether it is the stag or my husband, and he is tossed up into the air several times turning round. I go for help. My husband had been suffering pre-menstrual couvade with swelling hydration, irritability, hyperacuity of hearing and touch, toothache, lack of concentration, depression.'

A sooty chimney was the woman's dream on this last day of her cycle.

Another woman had a typical last day dream: 'Passing from threshold of several doors. A bathroom – I have a bath before passing through. I have a bath with J, a school-friend who menstruated earlier than I did.'

Another dreamer in a thirty-three-day cycle drinks the ovulation milk and approaches 'The House of the Dead' which is how ovulation sees the menstrual womb – maybe a festive event after all: 'I am late for rehearsal. The orchestra plays Elgar, Gerontius. They end as I walk up the corridor, with a pint of milk in my hand from which I am drinking. I apologize to the conductor for missing rehearsal. He smiles and says, next week we do "From the House of the Dead". Then the orchestra hall is set with tables for the dinner and dance. Lillian is there, she is writing Anglo Saxon riddles.'

In a longish cycle pre-menstrual hydration is imaged: 'I get out an old pink tracksuit with boots attached and there is water still in the boot from getting caught in the rain ages ago. I tip it out and then put boot to dry, explaining what I'm doing to my mother. I'd forgotten how nice a tracksuit it was and think I don't need to buy a new one.'

It is this woman's last day before her period: 'Biting through to other Queen, other self.'

And another has a late ovulation transition with loss followed by transformation of the dream child: 'My daughter is lying on mossy grass. I think she has been injured, run over by a bus. She lies back passively, her lower clothes are missing or pulled down and her legs covered with blood. She is fading, I see her sex open, pouring with blood. "It is my period," she says in a sort of gasp.' As if to say 'my period too', the daughter is just beginning her scanty periods.

The young menstrual animus approaches this woman, and is spurned with pre-menstrual anger: 'Outside is a slummy garden. I am putting out bulging, spilling-out garbage sacks, dog-shit on them. Several small boys about ten or eleven years old are playing with my daughter in the garden. The kids are noisy and grubby, local kids. I don't like them. The biggest boy is part black, with sallowy brown skin. I curse them. Get away, you fucking kids, I shout at them. They go away, the coloured boy looks defiant and sad. I feel bad about sending them away but can't put the rubbish out otherwise. I come back into the house, where all is lovely.'

DAY 29

Another dream by a woman in transition, with a pre-menstrual 'all-change': 'Trains. On a crowded train or bus giving a baby back to people. Then outside a dark wall by the sea, walking on top of it, talking to people, dark blowy place.'

This woman undergoes a particularly auspicious transition: 'Of being in a beautiful house, very small, we are in the kitchen. Everywhere are delightful beautiful objects, mostly kitchen utensils, old-fashioned, but lovely, not like a museum. I am very happy and look at everything in delight. This has either been left to us by an old kindly couple or we've bought it. They've made many of the things in here.

'Had a waking dream while the therapist was telling me about the birth trauma and its blood, of a lovely smell and the placenta floating made of the same substance as the wind. I used to talk to the moon when I was adolescent and said to it, "When, oh when is my period coming." Not long ago I found my daughter doing exactly the same thing.' This transition was made with full waking imagery and strong solidarity established both with her daughter and her past self.

DAY 30
Last day of cycle. Woman's daughter dreams of kitchen appliances working by themselves; husband dreams of a big electrical generating station.

This was a woman's dream of the period almost come: 'In a florist's. I buy some anemones, a small bunch. I say to the woman, how nice it is today. She says, this morning, early, everything was frozen solid. I open my purse, two pieces of pink ham fall out, then two tampons. I smile at the woman and fumble for a 50 pence piece.'

A man dreamed of the period nearly arrived and the womb-cone warming the room: 'A man in a box is thumping on the glass with the black stump of his severed hand. I daren't look at it. He bangs so hard the glass bulges. Then he is out – but not so menacing, and he has a cold. An oil fire warms the room, and we sit round it. It is the kind with gauze cone, which glows red-hot. I remember dreaming that image before, pre-menstrually: then it was a cone coming out of the earth like a small volcano that lighted the night up.'

DAY 31
The 'crime' of ovulation's death may well haunt a dreamer until the last day: 'I have killed a political leader in Yugoslavia (or similar place). I have shot him. I worry there will be fingerprints on gun. No one suspects me as I am good friend (girlfriend) of the murdered man.

'I am far away from the crime. I am in a country place, I'm outside in a lane, there are green hills and fields. A man comes to talk

APPENDIX

to me about the death. I am afraid, guilty, but I think no one suspects me.'

DAY 1
Transition achieved.

Woman: 'I dream that my best schoolfriend has started her period. When I wake up, my bleeding has begun. It is only my third time. I am glad it has come.'

Man: 'As the oriental man gives me the cup he looks straight into my eyes and says "This is my blood" and I feel a sharp physical pang within, as though the god is present.'

Notes

Introduction
1. Shuttle and Redgrove (1994), p.42.
2. Judith Higginbottom in Shuttle and Redgrove (1994), p.287.

1. The Joy of Dreaming
1. Fisher et al. (1983).
2. Benedek and Rubenstein (1939); Nagy-Bond (1966); Nagy (1981); Severino et al. (1989).
3. Zeller (1975), pp.158–63.
4. Mallon (1987), pp.56–7 and Chapter 3 passim.
5. Benedek and Rubenstein (1939).
6. Campbell (1968), figure on p.245; Walker (1983), pp.645–8.
7. Ulanov (1971), pp.46–50. Jung (1963), para 558, says: 'We take our stand simply and solely on the facts, recognising that the archetypal structure of the unconscious will produce over and over again and irrespective of tradition, those figures which reappear in the history of all epochs and all peoples, and will endow them with the same significance and numinosity that have been theirs from the beginning.' For Jung's puzzlement with blood, see Shuttle and Redgrove (1994), pp.315ff., note 3. In Jung (1963), para 690, he wonders whether the alchemist uses actual blood: 'Could it have been the adepts?' Indeed it could, if she were a woman.

2. The Road of Trials
1. In particular, Leviticus 15:19–30; 18:19; 20:18.
2. Shuttle and Redgrove (1994) Chapter 6.
3. Nagy-Bond (1966).

3. Dream-blood
1. Wilson (1976), p.81.

4. The Menstrual Mandala
1. O'Neill (1976), p.13.
2. Walker (1983), pp.645–8.
3. Wilson (1976), p.81.

6. Some Warnings and Encouragements
1. Shuttle and Redgrove (1994), pp.306–7.
2. A tableau in the Witch Museum at Boscastle, Cornwall, depicts the 'tar baby' practice vividly.
3. Ulanov (1971), discussion of animus, pp.41 ff.
4. Frazer (1913), Part One, Vol. 1, pp.8–9.
5. Harding (1955), p.62.
6. See note 7 to Chapter 1 for Jung's puzzlement over blood in alchemy.
7. Benedek and Rubenstein (1939).
8. Shuttle and Redgrove (1994), p.96.

7. Men and Menstruation
1. Knight (1991); Shuttle and Redgrove (1994), pp.70–2.
2. Fodor (1949).
3. Ulanov (1971), Part III, passim.
4. Knight (1991) gives a magnificent account of aboriginal menstruation and male menstrual customs, and shows how under certain conditions the men can ritually menstruate in harmony with the women.
5. Shuttle and Redgrove (1994), pp.276–9.
6. Ibid., p.187.

8. Moon and Weather
1. Murchie (1979), pp.178 ff.
2. Redgrove (1989), p.58. For data on weather sensitivity, pp.78 ff.
3. Patten and Patten (1988) is a useful on-going summary, but they warn that before you use the circuit with more than one person in it, you should consult Eeman (1947). They say that healing by laying on of hands is particularly effective with one subject in the circuit and the healer not connected up.

Very occasionally you get a person reacting as if the relaxation circuit were a tension circuit – one simply reverses the grips.
4. Patten and Patten (1988) give directions for quite elaborate silk and cotton circuits, but we have found silk strips for the hand connections and folded silk for the head and pelvis quite effective.

9. A Note on Rhythm
1. Schwenk (1965), p.30 – a beautifully illustrated book on the origin of natural rhythms, recommended for right-brain thoughts.
2. Murchie (1962), p.463.

10. Discarding the Negative
1. Harrison (1987), especially pp.34–5, 41–3, 135, 141–2.

11. Brain Opposites
1. Ornstein (1972), pp.70–1.
2. Ibid., p.69.
3. Edwards (1988), passim: Sewell (1960), passim.
4. Durden-Smith and deSimone (1983), pp.51–67: see also Moir and Jessel (1989), pp.17–20, 107, on the sensory differences between men and women.
5. Gooch (1972).
6. Shuttle and Redgrove (1994), p.93.

14. Rites of Passage
1. The basic book is still Gennep (1960).

15. A Useful Waking-dream Technique
1. Wilson (1976), p.81.

16. Yoga and its Analogues
1. Redgrove (1989), p.201, note 91.
2. Long (1981).
3. Walker (1983), p.821; 'Menstrual Blood', 'Prostitution' *passim*.
4. Pearsall (1989), p.xvi and passim.
5. Gauld (1992), pp.11 ff.

6. Douglas and Slinger (1979). 'Four Joys', pp.192–4; 'Riding the Waves of Ecstasy', pp.145–6.
7. Redgrove (1989), p.175.

17. Homoeopathy, Hypnosis, Acupuncture and Massage
1. The description of Do-In massage is only a sketch. Rofidal (1981) is recommended. The massage spiral is summarized on p.46.

Afterword
1. Fisher et al. (1983).
2. Wilson (1976), p.81.

Bibliography of Works Cited

ALLEN, Paula Gunn (1986). *The Sacred Hoop.* Boston: Beacon Press.
BENEDEK, Therese and RUBENSTEIN, Boris B. (1939). 'The Correlations between Ovarian Activity and Psychodymanic Processes: 1. The Ovulative Phase', *Psychosomatic Medicine,* Vol. 1, No. 2, pp.245–70; 2. The Menstrual Phase, Vol. 1, No. 4, pp.461–85.
CAMPBELL, Joseph (1968). *The Hero With a Thousand Faces.* New York: Princeton University Press, Bollingen Series XVII.
DOUGLAS, Nik and SLINGER, Penny (1979). *Sexual Secrets: the Alchemy of Ecstasy.* London: Hutchinson.
DURDEN-SMITH, Jo and deSIMONE, Diane (1983). *Sex and the Brain.* London: Pan Books.
EDWARDS, Betty (1988). *Drawing on the Right Side of the Brain.* London: Fontana/Collins.
EEMAN, L. E. (1947). *Co-operative Healing: The Curative Properties of Human Radiations.* London: Muller.
FISHER, C. et al. (1983). 'Patterns of Female Sexual Arousal during Sleep and Waking', *Archives of Sexual Behaviour,* Vol. 12, pp.97–122.
FRAZER, J. G. (1913). *The Golden Bough.* London: Macmillan.
FODOR, Nandor (1949). *The Search for the Beloved.* New York: University Books.
GAULD, Alan (1992). *A History of Hypnotism.* Cambridge: CUP.
GENNEP, A. Van (1960). *The Rites of Passage.* London: Routledge and Kegan Paul.
GOOCH, Stan (1972). *Total Man: Notes towards an Evolutionary Theory of Personality.* London: Allen Lane, The Penguin Press.

BIBLIOGRAPHY

HARDING, M. Esther (1955). *Woman's Mysteries.* New York: Pantheon.
HARRISON, Michelle (1987). *Self-Help with PMS.* London: Optima/Macdonald.
JUNG, C. G. (1963). *Mysterium Conjunctionis,* Vol. 14 of Collected Works. London: Routledge and Kegan Paul.
KNIGHT, Chris (1991). *Blood Relations: Menstruation and the Origins of Culture.* New Haven and London: Yale University Press.
LONG, Mary (1981). 'Visions of a New Force', *Science Digest,* Vol. 89, Part 10, pp.36–42.
MALLON, Brenda (1987). *Women Dreaming.* London: Fontana.
MOIR, Anne and JESSEL, David (1989). *Brainsex.* London: Michael Joseph.
MORRIS, Jan (1974). *Conundrum.* London: Faber and Faber.
MURCHIE, Guy (1962). *Music of the Spheres.* London: Secker and Warburg.
MURCHIE, Guy (1979). *The Seven Mysteries of Life: An Exploration in Science and Philosophy.* London: Rider/ Hutchinson.
NAGY, M. (1981). 'Menstruation and Shamanism', *Psychological Perspectives,* Vol. 12, Part I, pp.52–68.
NAGY-BOND, Marilyn (1966). 'Menstruation and Psychic Maturity', essay submitted to C. G. Jung Institute in partial fulfilment of requirements for analyst's diploma.
O'NEIL, W. N. (1976). *Time and the Calendars.* Manchester: Manchester University Press.
ORNSTEIN, Robert, E. (1972). *The Psychology of Consciousness.* San Francisco: W. H. Freeman.
PATTEN, Leslie, with PATTEN, Terry (1988). *Biocircuits.* California: H. J. Kramer.
PEARSALL, Paul (1989). *Super Marital Sex.* London: Futura/ Macdonald.
PERRY, George (1987). *The Complete Phantom of the Opera.* London: Pavilion.
REDGROVE, Peter (1989). *The Black Goddess and the Sixth Sense.* London: Paladin Grafton Books.
ROFIDAL, Jean (1981). *Do-In.* Wellingborough: Thorson.
ROSSI, Ernest (1977). 'The Cerebral Hemispheres in Analytical Psychology', *Journal of Analytical Psychology,* Vol. 22, No. 1.

SCHWENK, Theodore (1965). *Sensitive Chaos*. London: Rudolph Steiner Press.

SEVERINO, Sally K. et al. (1989). 'Cyclical Changes in Emotional Information Processing in Sleep and Dreams', *Journal of the American Academy of Psychoanalysis*, Vol. 17, No. 4, pp.555–77.

SEWELL, Elizabeth (1960). *The Orphic Voice*. London: Routledge and Kegan Paul.

SHUTTLE, Penelope, and REDGROVE, Peter (1994). *The Wise Wound: Menstruation and Everywoman*. London: HarperCollins.

ULANOV, Ann Belford (1971). *The Feminine in Jungian Psychology and in Christian Theology*. Evanston: Northwestern University Press.

WALKER, Barbara G. (1983). *The Women's Encyclopedia of Myths and Secrets*. San Francisco: Harper and Row.

WILSON, Frank Avray (1976). *Alchemy as a Way of Life*. London: C. W. Daniel.

ZELLER, Max (1975). *The Dream – The Vision of the Night*. The Analytical Psychology Club of Los Angeles and the C. G. Jung Institute of Los Angeles.

Index

Page numbers in *italic* refer to the illustrations

'abominable meal' dream, 20–1
aborigines, 70
acupuncture, 148
Agni, 59
Allen, Paula Gunn, 7
anal contractions, 131
animals, 112, 129
animus, 46–52, 54–63, 125
ankh, 59, 106
archetypes, 15, 155
aromatherapy, 44, 109, 128
art, creativity, 94–5
aspirin, 83
Assagioli, Roberto, 99
Asvini mudra, 139
autonomic nervous system, 104
autoscopy, 78

Bach Rescue Remedy, 147
bandhas, 139–40
Benedek, Therese, 11, 13, 62, 63
birth, 23–4, 66–7, 72
Black Goddess, 23, 60
blood, 20, 23, 25, 66–7, 109
see also menstruation
brain, 'left' and 'right', 96–105

breast-feeding, 69
breathing, 83, 128, 130–2, 149, 152

calendar, 31–3, 79
'calling each other down', 121–6
Campbell, Joseph, 13, 67
Catholic Church, 46
cerebellum, 104
ceremonies, 119
cervix, 34, 44–5, 72
Charles, Prince of Wales, 10, 26, 27
children:
 in dreams, 47
 and menstrual rhythm, 70, 110
Christianity, 101–2, 111
churches, 111
circulatio, 35
clairvoyance, 41
clitoris, 20, 57, 59–60, 137
clothes, 124, 143
comedians, 55–7
convergers, 104–5
cooking, 129
corpus luteum, 60, 72, 73, 92, 114, 117
couvade, 50, 68, 73

creativity, 92–5, 107, 132
cross, looped, 59
crux ansata, 59, 60
cyclical time, 31–3, 71–2

dampness, 85
dark man, 22
Death-in-Life, 125
dehumidifiers, 85
Descartes, René, 90
Diana, Princess of Wales, 26
divergers, 104–5
Do-In, 83, 149–50
Dr Jekyll and Mr Hyde, 54
'double pelican', 43, *117*, 118
dream-creatures, 43–4
dreams:
    enjoyment of, 9–11
    and the immune system, 147
    luteal phase, 62
    men's, 10, 19, 73, 154
    in menstrual cycle, 1–2, 5–6, 11–28, 154
    menstruation, 18, 25–8, 62, 63, 157–9
    nightmares, 39–40
    ovulation, 12–14, 17–18, 25, 62, 160–3
    and PMS, 4–5
    in pre-menstrual state, 18, 22–4, 62–3, 163–9
    recording, 38
    recurring, 49, 50–1
    redreaming, 61
    rhythm, 38–45
    and sexuality, 60, 135, 156
    sharing, 43, 66, 71
    stimulating, 43
    waking dreams, 121–6

dysmenorrhoea, 105, 109, 120, 131

Edwards, Betty, 102
Eeman circuits, 85–6
Egypt, 47, 59, 60
ejaculation, 139, 140
electricity, sensitivity to, 81, 82, 83–4
Elizabeth II, Queen, 10, 27
Ellis, Havelock, 13, 63
Elton, Ben, 55
'empty nest' syndrome, 3
erotic living, 141
excremental images, 19–20
exercise, 127, 139
expectations, 91–5

falling dreams, 19
feet, reflexology, 149
fetishism, 143–4
fish symbol, 14
Fodor, Nandor, 67
Franz, Marie Louise von, 13
Frazer, Sir James, 52–3
French, Dawn, 55–7, 60
Freud, Sigmund, 79

gardening, 111, 129
Golden Dawn, 64
Gooch, Stan, 104
Graafian follicle, 114

handedness, left and right, 96–7, 98–9
Harding, Esther, 57–9
Harrison, Dr Michelle, 91–2, 93, 94
Hatha yoga, 129–30, 138
headaches, 130, 150

headstands, 129–30
Henry, Lenny, 55
Hillman, James, 145
Holy Ghost, 111
homoeopathy, 44, 83, 146–7
hormones, 60, 128, 156
   divergers and convergers, 105
   and dysmenorrhoea, 109
   falling dreams, 19
   fluctuations in men, 70
   menstrual cycle, 16, 114
   ovulation, 17
   pheromones, 71, 89, 94, 128, 155
   and sex of foetus, 67
   and sexuality, 72
   testosterone arousal, 136
horror films, 62–3
houses, in dreams, 19
humidity, 85
hydration, 17, 82, 94
hypnosis, 147–8
hysterectomy, 3

I Ching, 117, 118
illness, pre-menstrual magnification (PMM), 93–4
illogic, 102–3, 106
immune system, 44, 147
ionizers, 84
Isis, 47, 59, 106–7

jalandhara bandha, 140
Jesus, 53, 111
jet-lag, 90
jewels, dreams of, 12, 13
Jews, 46
Jung, C.G., 60–2, 134

Kelly, Robert, 75
King Kong, 53

language:
   brain lateralization, 102, 103–4
   sealed writing, 144–5
'left brain', 96–105, 107
lesbians, 94
Life-in-Death, 125
light, 84
linear time, 31, 71
logic, 102–3
looped cross, 59, 106
'lucid' dreams, 78
lunar time, 31, 33
luteal phase:
   dreams, 62
   sexuality, 138

magic, 64
Mallon, Brenda, 12, 13–14
Mamoulian, Rouben, 54
mandala, menstrual, 2, 31–7, 32, 42, 43, 53, 71, 79–80, 125–6, 135, 142
Marsh, Fredric, 54
Mary Magdalen, 102, 111
masculine tradition, 52–3
massage, 131, 148–50
masturbation, 20, 59, 60, 70, 144
meditation, 127–8
men:
   anima, 51
   couvade, 50
   dreams, 10, 19, 73, 154
   initiation cycle, 67–8
   'left brain' and 'right brain', 98–100

    and menstruation, 66–73
    sexuality, 72, 132–5, 136–40, 142–4
    yoga, 130
menopause, 154
menstrual cycle:
    dreaming in, 2, 5–6, 11–28, 154
    expectations, 91–5
    and the moon, 58, 79
    pre-menstrual state, 3–4
    rhythm, 87–90
    rites of passage, 119–20
    and sexuality, 129, 132, 135–6
    synchrony, 89, 94, 110, 128
'menstrual kit', 108
menstrual mandala, 31–7, *32*, 42, 43, 53, 71, 79–80, 125–6, 135, 142
menstruation, 2, 11–12
    animus, 46–8
    attitudes to, 3–4
    conflict with ovulation, 15
    dreams, 18, 25–8, 62, 63, 157–9
    first period, 20, 119
    'left brain' and 'right brain', 96–103
    men and, 66–73
    and the moon, 79
    and sexuality, 129, 132, 135, 136, 137
Mesmer, Anton, 86, 141
minerals, 69
moon, 31, 37, 58, 79–80, 87–8, 106, 117, 118
Morris, Jan, 133–4
mother images, 22
mula bandha, 139

Murchie, Guy, 77
museums, 111
musicals, 53

Nagy-Bond, Marilyn, 23
negative expectations, 91–5
negative ions, 83–4
Nightmare on Elm Street, 54–5
nightmares, 39–40
nose, alternate nostril breathing, 130–1

oestrogen, 19, 105, 114, 116
O'Neill, Professor W.M., 31–3
oral sex, 109
orgasm, 59, 60, 120, 121, 129, 131, 132–3, 135, 137–8, 139–41
oscillators, 88–9
ovarian cycle, 114, *115*, *116*, 117–18
ovulation, 2, 11
    animus, 48
    conflict with menstruation, 15
    dreams, 12–14, 17–18, 25, 62, 160–3
    'left brain' and 'right brain', 96–103
    men and, 71
    pre-ovulation syndrome (POS), 4, 68, 120
    and sexuality, 129, 132, 135–6
    signs of, 34
'ovulation kit', 108
ovum, 114

paraphilias, 142–4

INDEX

pelvic floor exercises, 131
Peredur, 57
The Phantom of the Opera, 48, 53–4
pheromones, 71, 89, 94, 128, 155
photographs, 107
placebo effect, 5, 119
Plath, Sylvia, 101
poetry, 101, 102, 142
polarity healing, 85–6
polarity massage, 150
pranayama, 131–2
pre-menstrual magnification (PMM), 93–4
pre-menstrual state, 3–4
  dreams, 18, 22–4, 62–3, 163–9
  senses, 78
  and sexuality, 136
pre-menstrual syndrome (PMS):
  animus dreams, 49–50
  couvade, 68
  and dreams, 4–5
  as medical problem, 3, 4
  stages of, 72, 120
  symptoms, 3
pre-ovulation syndrome (POS), 4–5, 68, 120
Prescott, James, 133
progesterone, 16, 17, 19, 72, 105, 114, 117
prostaglandins, 60, 128
puberty, 155

reflexology, 149
relaxation, 43, 61, 127, 138–9, 151–3
religion, 124–5, 133

Rescue Remedy, 147
rhythm, 87–90, 120
'right brain', 4, 96–105, 106, 107
rites of passage, 119–20
'room of one's own', 107–8
Rubenstein, Boris, 11, 62, 63

scarab, 12–13
science, 98, 101, 135
sealed writing, 43, 144–5
Seasonal Affective Disorder (SAD), 84
Sekhmet, 41, 56, 58, 59
semen, 109
senses, 77–8
serotonin, 90
Sewell, Elizabeth, 102
sexuality, 72, 128–9, 132–44, 156
sharing dreams, 43, 66, 71
shark images, 23
shiatsu, 148
shoulderstands, 129–30
'sixth sense', 83
skin, 150
sleep, 110, 151
smells, 108–9
'sniffles', 94
Stevenson, R.L., 54
stimulating dreams, 43
symbols, 106–7, 118
synchrony, menstrual cycles, 89, 94, 110, 128

T'ai Chi, 139
Tantrism, 142
Taoist yoga, 138
Tarot, 118
Tat cross, 106–7

temperature, 34–5
Terrible Mother, 22, 23
testosterone, 70, 71, 136, 154
time, 31–3
Tracy, Spencer, 54
transformation dreams, 21–2
trans-sexualism, 134
trees, 48, 57, 60
turn-ons, 143

Ulanov, Ann Belford, 15, 48–9, 67
'vacuum headache', 130
vibrations, water, 87–8
Virgin Mary, 101–2, 111
vitamin B6, 4
vitamins, 69

waking dreams, 121–6
Walker, Barbara G., 13, 33, 133
walking, 110–11, 139

water:
  dreams of, 14–15
  vibrations, 87–8
weather sensitivity, 78, 80–5, 132
wheel cross, 79, 80, 118
whole-breathing, 131–2
Wiccans, 58
Williams, Robin, 55
Wilson, Frank Avray, 156
Wisewoman Cycle, 58
witches, 21, 47–8, 62, 80, 111, 155
womb, 80
womb-cycle, 114–18, *115*, *116*
Woolf, Virginia, 101, 107–8
writing, sealed, 43, 144–5

Yeats, W.B., 134
Yin-Yang, 117, 118
yoga, 83, 127–32, 138, 139

Zeller, Max, 12